TO LOSE WEIGHT NATURALLY IS TO

# Believe in it!

**How to Harness the Power of Your Mind to Lose Weight, Stay Healthy, and Feel Better About Your Inner Self**

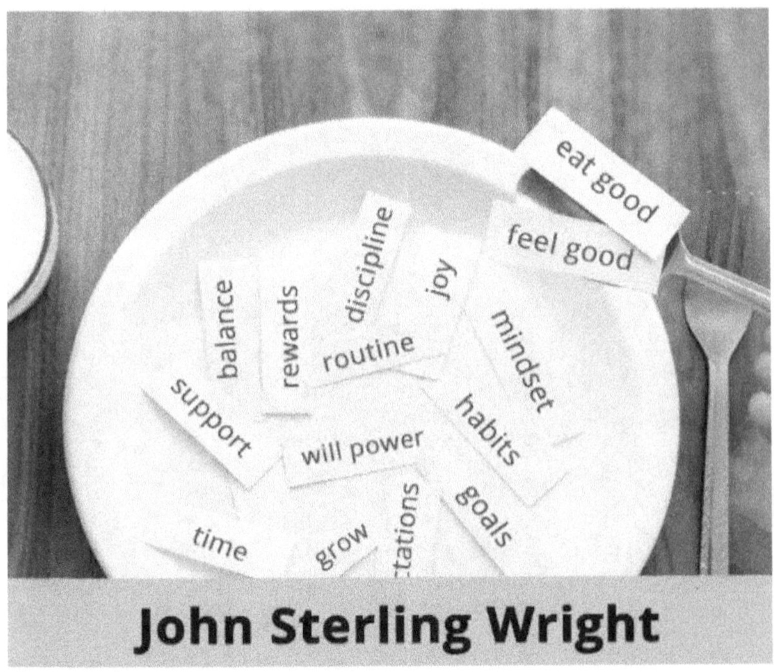


## John Sterling Wright

# John Sterling Wright

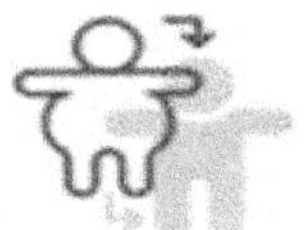

Copyright © 2022 John Wright

All rights reserved.

All rights reserved. No part of this book may be reproduced or used in any manner without the prior written permission of the copyright owner, except for the use of brief quotations in a book review.

# Table of Contents:

An escape from sure death came on suddenly at age 55…Heart Attack! The kind the doctor called the widow maker. But how could this be, I wasn't that old yet and still had a 12-year-old son to raise, being a single dad, and bringing up my boy from when he was a baby all on my own. As I lay there in the ER with the cardiologist on duty asking me all these different questions, one in particular really hit home, "do you smoke" the doctor asked, and I replied yes. He said, "not anymore, being overweight and smoking are two of the biggest reasons that led you here today." So, I quit right then and there after hearing those chilling words from the doctor, and it was easier than I thought it would be.

After my recovery from the surgery, I knew that I had to make changes in my life for the good, and so, I had a come to Jesus moment with myself, being honest with my inner self about all the negative things that brought me to this moment. I knew I had to come up with a solution to all my problems so I could be around to see my son graduate from high school and college. So, I did a lot of research and studied for years about all the aspects of weight loss, health/diet, and how the mind works that affect all of the different aspects of both, and also the rest of your goals in life. And, how to reset my way of thinking, (mindset), that I needed to change the negative things in my life that were hindering me in my thought process about different things in life that I wanted to accomplish but hadn't. I read many books and articles by the top experts in the fields of weight loss, diet/nutrition, health, mindset, and physical fitness, studying all of them very carefully. I took notes and put them in writing so that if I had a moment of hesitation or doubt, it was there right in front of me. This I did to reinforce my way of thinking and keep on track to create a positive mindset that I could put to use to accomplish all of that. And, all the notes I wrote down and studying I did, is how this book came to be.

If you are one of the many people out there that has tried in the past to lose weight, I know your pain. You might be one of the ones that have tried dieting plans that promise to melt the pounds away, like Jenny Craig, weight watchers, the Keto diet, etc. And you might have some success in losing weight quickly, but these are what most people turn to when summer swimsuit season comes around, a wedding to go to, or a class reunion, and so on. But all they are really, are just hollow shallow promises that over a period of time, people tend to stop because they have accomplished what they wanted to do for a short span, and they revert back to the old ways and put back on the weight they might have lost, and then some. They are costly to maintain for a long time, which is one reason people give up on them. In their own minds, they reason that now I can gain a few pounds and I will still look good. They create a state of denial in that way of thinking, and never follow through with anything else in life, which is to make the positive changes needed to stay mentally strong and healthy. A strong mentality is the first and most important thing to having success with the rest of the goals you set out to accomplish, especially in losing weight. Diet and exercise of course play an important role in all of this too. Without the three of them combined you will not have much or any success.

I know my plan was the key to my turnaround for a healthier lifestyle, and a more positive way of thinking that led to a happier, more self-confident me. I was able to turn my life around for the better and haven't looked back since. I quit smoking cold turkey, lost the excess weight, (32lbs), and have kept it off for the past 15 years now, and so can you! Follow in my footsteps as I lead you on the journey to creating the mindset you need to succeed in losing weight, staying healthy, and having a strong self-assurance going forward in life, which has worked very well for me and I know it will work for you too!

I'm going to share with you the building blocks for a strong mentality that are of the utmost importance when it comes to weight loss. This is where you start to construct your foundation towards a positive outcome for a more self-confident you. By doing so, losing weight is easy and so is everything else in life that you set out to accomplish.

In this book, I will show you how to put it all together, so it becomes a daily routine that is easy for you to follow and stick to. So, let's do this thing, and take the plunge and dive right in, in your quest for a better, healthier, and happier you!

I'm writing this book for two reasons. First, I want to share with you a way to lose weight and to keep it off so you too can see a healthy transformation and be able to enjoy life again. It's not that fad diets like the keto diet, Jenny Craig's model, Weight Watchers, and the likes don't work. They do, and they're quite potent. In fact, throughout this book, I will be referring to them. The problem with all of them is that they are short-term solutions to a long-term problem. They're geared toward being able to drop a load of weight quickly so you can fit into a wedding dress, go on vacation, or just to get back into that swimsuit and be able to look and feel great again.

Here's a sobering statistic: 90% of dieters gain back the pounds they had worked so hard to lose. Can we blame the weight loss regime for that? No, we can't. There must be another reason. I believe the answer is found in what we eat and how we deal with life outside of our weight loss goals. A holistic approach to weight loss must also include a strong mental state. Our mind's attitude toward food is a big part of this picture but what else is missing? I'll get to that shortly.

It's not just the fad diets, it's our own mindset toward food and life in general that leaves us confused and empty. It's a mess we didn't create by ourselves. Society in general created the mess we are now all caught up in. Why is the color red so prominent in many fast-food logos? Wendy's, Burger King, McDonald's, KFC, Pizza Hut etc. Why is it that everything we see is colorfully, bright red? The word red seems to permeate our subconscious minds. Consumerism has conditioned us to see red with food everywhere we go. Before you even realize it, your subconscious mind is sending signals to your body that it's time to eat and the hunger pangs begin. This is only one of the many ways we are tempted on a daily basis in this overstimulated world of today.

Secondly, I want to share with you how to transform this unhealthy mindset into something positive and useful for your life's journey. I'll give you step-by-step directions on how to change your thoughts about food, eating, and taking care of yourself in general. I'll help you learn the tricks of the trade so that when you feel that need for a delicious, indulgent treat, you can say no without guilt or remorse. Then I'll take it a step further by helping you devise a plan of action that includes small healthy changes that eventually add up to big results. Weight loss should be slow and steady. Then it's easy to maintain. I'll show you how to change your mindset so you can stay on the right track and never give up. Most importantly, I'll help you develop a healthy relationship with food and eating by including the activities that will naturally keep your weight down low and your outlook positive for a healthier and happier life for yourself in the near future.

Are you ready to begin a fun and exciting journey? Are you ready to discover the serendipitous benefits of an improved mindset while you are dramatically changing your body? Good! It's time to begin. Let's do this!

# About The Author -- Who Is John Wright

John Wright is a single father that has had a battle with weight loss, eating healthy, and exercising in the past. He has been overweight most of his adult life having tried many different diets and exercises that never worked because of a lack of commitment.

After the frightening experience in the ER, which was a real eye-opener, enabled him to change his life around for the good. He has researched and studied for years the teachings of many of the top experts in the fields of nutrition, weight loss, health, physical fitness, and different aspects of developing a positive mindset that it takes to accomplish all of your goals in life in life that have eluded you so far. Nowadays he's healthy, happy, and physically fit, and enjoys the life he is living. He's from Chino Valley, Arizona, where he spends his free time outdoors riding the back roads in the country around him and taking in the sights and scenes that nature has to offer. He's also an avid arts and crafts enthusiast.

## What this book is about

Why do we pay for gym memberships and then don't go? Why comfort ourselves with a pint of ice cream knowing we'll regret it the next day? How can we harness the power of our mind to lose weight, stay healthy and feel better about our inner selves? Believing is the answer!

In "Believe In It!" you'll learn how to change your lifestyle and bolster your mindset so you can
finally start losing weight. You'll see that losing weight and staying healthy, enjoying delicious
meals, and feeling good about your inner self is possible. Diets are a temporary fix and not a real solution. People who are successful in losing weight are those who have  power of the mind. In this book you'll learn how to:

- Change your lifestyle to lose weight, and feel healthy, and good about yourself.

- Stop being your own worst enemy when it comes to losing weight.

- Manage stress and prevent it from aggravating your health; And much more!

In this book, you will get a complete understanding of what you need to change, where to start, and, how to accomplish all of this in a 3-step methodology that put into practice will change your life forever! So, climb aboard the train and see where it takes you on a journey to all the possibilities of what your life has to offer.

# Who is this book for?

Maybe you're feeling hopeless, angry, or resentful. Maybe you're feeling inspired, determined, or proud. Whatever the case may be, these feelings are trying to tell you that your life would improve if you started acting in a certain way. This book is for those of us who:


- Have ever started a weight loss diet and failed to reach our goals?


When we feel discouraged, it's easy to blame the diet or program we were following. We may decide that we're doomed to be overweight forever. This is a faulty belief that will only lead to more discouragement and failure. When we fall off the wagon, we're usually too embarrassed to admit it. Instead, we offer excuses or rationalizations that convince ourselves that losing weight wasn't worth the effort. It's easier not to try again than it is to admit failure.


- Have ever felt criticized by others because of our weight?


Some people enjoy pointing out our weight problems as if we're not aware of them or as if it's our fault for being overweight. In reality, we're all victims of a society that encourages overeating by bombarding us with unhealthy food choices everywhere we go. For many years, I walked around in a fog knowing why I was so heavy but couldn't figure out a way to change it.

- Are looking for a change that's long overdue.

There is no time like the present to make positive changes in your life. Get out of the way of your own success by giving up those 'what if' thoughts and start living life! Use dieting as a tool to guide you on your journey rather than as a crutch. There's only one way to fix your weight problem—through diet and exercise along with other healthy habits. I encourage you to break free of the chains that have held you back for so long. Make good choices today so you can succeed when it counts.

- Are tired of making New Year's Resolutions and then giving up on them.

Why wait for the New Year to start a diet? It's time to make the changes that will give you the healthy lifestyle you deserve. You deserve to live your best life and have a positive attitude about yourself and your health. Put an end to being overweight by changing your thoughts about food, eating, and exercising. Saying no to bad habits is only one step on your journey to a slimmer you!

By following the techniques in this book, you will:

- Feel confident about your ability to change.

- Feel proud about the progress you've made.

- Be able to make decisions that will improve your relationship with food, eating, and yourself.

- Be able to identify those unhealthy thoughts which will make you want to overeat.

- Take the first step in making positive changes for a healthier and happier life.

Most importantly, and I've saved the best for last, you will see a sustainable lifestyle that will help you lose weight. It isn't so tough that you'll feel deprived. You will feel inspired and empowered to make the right choices for your success. Let's start this weight loss journey together!

# Introduction

**Acting against our better judgment**

There should be a word for that familiar feeling we have when we know that we should be doing something but can't get ourselves to do it. It's not procrastination, laziness, or a lack of motivation. It's something else that is more challenging to explain, but just as difficult to escape from. If you feel it, you know it. This word does actually exist, and it's called akrasia.

This feeling is especially strong when we're about to do something that requires effort, commitment, and hard work. The reason we can't get started is because we've been programmed by society to believe that what we are about to do will be painful, difficult, or unpleasant in some way.

All of these feelings are enough to put off even the most determined soul. Sometimes it impedes us from doing things we'd like to do simply because we can't get started; and so, we find it more convenient to do nothing.

Akrasia is a hindrance that can hold us back from experiencing a happier and more productive life if we don't learn how to overcome it. The best way to overcome akrasia is to know that you're susceptible to this feeling and then alert yourself in time to stop procrastinating and get the ball rolling.


When Steve Maraboli said that "It's not just about losing the weight; it's about losing the lifestyle and mindset that got you there" he had realized that his life was out of control and had to change. He believed that he needed to create a new vision for himself and his future that included losing weight, rather than resorting to doing it for everyone else.

# CHAPTER 1:

# The power of the mind

In my opinion, the real secret to losing weight isn't in finding the "best" weight loss diet or hiring a personal trainer who can give you the "right" exercises for losing weight. What matters isn't something quantifiable. It's not a product, a routine, an app, or a system. It's simply a change in the way you think about food.

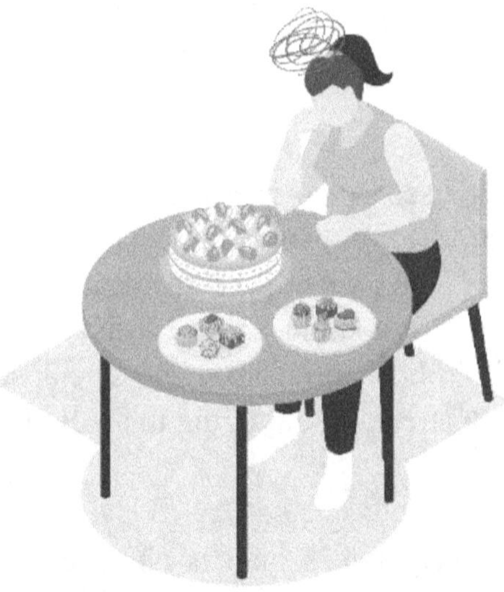

The modern diet industry is founded on the premise that we need to go to extreme measures to stop ourselves from eating. Things like setting an eating window, obsessively counting calories, self-starvation, and depriving ourselves of indulgences. While there is a time and place for these things (and I'll talk about that a little later on in chapter 4), if you're looking for the fastest, easiest, and healthiest way to lose weight, it starts with understanding that food is nourishment.

A healthy diet is not about "dieting". It's about learning to eat in a way that satisfies your body's needs while not compromising the things you love. Restrictive diets leave out taste and convenience, so you have to "think" about every morsel of food you eat. When a calorie-counting approach forces you to think about what you're eating, it pushes away the enjoyment that should come from eating.

The human body is a complex machine, and when you force it to work against its natural inclinations, you are setting yourself up for failure. Our willpower is finite. The more you rely on self-control, the less of it you have for other important things.

A "motivation-based" plan is usually not sustainable. If you rely on motivation to lose weight, what happens when your motivation fades? You gain back all the weight and perhaps even a few extra pounds for good measure. Motivation can be fleeting, and even if it isn't, how motivating can a relapse be when you break a two-week streak by indulging in an old favorite?

A sustainable weight loss plan is about eating more of the things you love when you're hungry, and less of the things that make you feel sick and tired.

There are several other reasons to avoid motivation-based weight loss plans. One of them is the concept of "All or Nothing Thinking". This cognitive distortion describes the idea that if you don't reach your goal perfectly, then you have failed. Perfectionism leads to cycles of self-loathing. You may have heard the term "Health at Every Size". It refers to a lifestyle where health and well-being are prioritized regardless of weight.

Healthy doesn't mean thin. Healthy doesn't even mean "in shape". What it does mean is being physically fit, which means you can do the things that life demands you do. If you need a quick snapshot of "health" that doesn't require an Olympic training regimen, simply stand up and see if you can touch your toes. If you can, then you are reasonably fit enough to be considered "healthy". We need to stop chasing the idea of thin and start chasing health.

**How our mindset affects our success in different areas of life**

It is not just weight loss which we are after, but it is also about positive thinking, finding the right goal, and sticking to it. The right mindset can be an important ingredient in achieving success. How we think about things can affect the way we feel, and how we feel affects the way we do things. A growth mindset is a belief that you can improve, and that intelligence and skills are not fixed but expandable. When comparing that to a fixed mindset, which is the idea that we are born with a certain amount of talent, ability, intelligence, or character; we see that a growth mindset helps us grow our skills and achieve greater results in everything we do. It can be a game changer for anyone who wants to achieve their goals.

Our health is one of the 8 pillars of holistic wellness. It is linked to our mental and spiritual well-being. By tackling the mindset first, we can see positive changes in our overall health and well-being. If we understand the why of it, then it is really easy to fit into our life.

## The role that mindset plays in achieving success

If we believe that we can achieve something and are determined to do so, it creates an internal energy that drives us to reach our goals. On the other hand, if we doubt ourselves and think that the odds are stacked against us, we will often become demotivated and give up. The trick is to change your mind set by creating a new perception of self. This way you can start seeing yourself as a person who is capable of achieving almost anything!

When we believe that we can do something, we set ourselves up for success. This is because the brain releases endorphins when we have a positive attitude and see things in a constructive way. It makes us feel good, gives us energy and increases our overall confidence. So if you believe that you are capable of achieving something, it becomes more than possible!

In order to develop a growth mindset and achieve your goals, start by changing your perception of self and your attitude. Believe that you can do it no matter the circumstances. Even if you don't always feel positive or optimistic right away, just keep going and reminding yourself that you are on the right track. This will become a self-fulfilling prophecy and your hard work will pay off in the end.

Our mindset impacts our self-esteem, perspective, drive, resilience and reality. When we believe that our efforts will eventually pay off, we are more likely to be persistent and stick with it. When we believe that we can overcome our challenges and succeed, it puts us in the right frame of mind for making positive changes in our life. It is a cycle of success where we start with a positive perception of ourselves and then build on it by doing the right things.

**When negative thinking hinders weight loss**

What holds us back from achieving our goals is often a negative mindset. We think about how difficult it will be to change our life or how we don't have enough time or energy to make the necessary changes. We then start blaming ourselves for not being able to get things right and that just creates more negativity. Studies have shown that a negative self-image sabotages our Weight loss efforts in a few interesting ways.

People who are dissatisfied with their bodies are likely to avoid exercising. Body dissatisfaction could be in the form of not liking our body, not feeling comfortable in your body or disliking certain parts of our bodies. It has been shown that people with a negative self-image will avoid physical activity because it enhances awareness of their bodies. The stigma of being overweight will make it hard to exercise in public and the negative thinking that the person with a negative self-image has will make them think that other people will judge them. In order to avoid scrutiny, they then avoid exercise.

Self-esteem in the form of liking your body is a key component to achieving weight loss. If we feel good about ourselves and our bodies, we are much more likely to be active when it comes to exercising. This is why people who have a very positive self-image who feel good about their body will be much more likely to exercise regularly and participate in physical activities.


-   Negative thinking leads to emotional eating.


Emotional eating is nothing but an attempt by the person affected to manage their emotions by using food. People who rely on emotional eating would be happier if they were to replace that bad habit with good habits like exercising, reading, or meditating. Studies have shown that people who rely on emotional eating when they are stressed, sad or angry, tend to indulge in calorie-dense comfort foods either late at night or in the morning as a pick-me-up after a sleepless night.


Pizza, chocolate, and ice cream top the list of comfort foods. Stress eating is an attempt to cope with negative emotions like anxiety, anger, and sadness. But it doesn't really work because we relearn the negative habits that we give in to in order to deal with our emotional state. This is a negative loop where we eat when we are in an emotional state and then feel bad about ourselves which makes us eat more. That turns into a vicious cycle of weight gain.


-   We're likely to gain weight when we think that we're overweight

In a 2015 study published in the International Journal of Obesity, researchers looked at how negative thoughts about our weight can affect how much we weigh. The results of the study were rather conclusive. Participants who were told that they were heavier than they actually were, lost less weight than those who had been told that they were lighter than they actually were. Their body image or self-image as a heavier person affected their eating habits and also their physical activity which hampered their weight loss efforts.

What we think affects how we feel, act and ultimately how much of a success we will be in losing weight. This is because our mindset is what gets hold of us and keeps us from reaching our goals. When we have negative thinking about our weight, we will inevitably find ourselves in a vicious cycle where we start eating more and exercising less. It is therefore crucial that we learn to take control of our minds so that we can achieve our weight loss goals.

- Positive self-talk is crucial to weight loss

That inner dialogue, or the continuous loop of thoughts that run through our heads, is called self-talk. Our lives are filled with a continuous stream of thoughts that run through our minds - many of them involve what we think about other people, our jobs, the weather, and yes...our body image. When we have a minor relapse on our weight loss journey, such as failing to meet a calorie count or skipping a day, positive self-talk has the power to turn our negative thought patterns into positive ones.

It keeps us motivated even when we are not getting the results that we want and expect. And we need it - as much as we need a sunny day. Without positive self-talk we can become so frustrated, so discouraged that we just give up.

We have all experienced those days when we are so frustrated, tired, and irritated that we just can't make the time to exercise. On those days our negative self-talk becomes too much of an inconvenience. Without positive self-talk we sit in front of the TV and let negative thoughts bombard us. We feel like everything is a bother - getting up in the morning, coming home from work, making dinner for our family and then exercising after that double cheeseburger. We get so ticked off that we finally decide to just let it all go - to just say "screw it" and turn on the TV.

By using affirmations, we can turn negative thoughts that drive us away from exercise into positive ones. Affirmations can help us create a new reality where exercise is an integral part of our life.

Affirmations can be short and simple, such as:

**I am strong**

**I am beautiful**

**I love my body**

or they can be long and involved, such as:

I have the strength to accomplish my goals, I accept myself as I am, including all of my imperfections, things will always get better if I keep trying and so on. They also make a great addition to positive self-talk scripts such as the following one: "I'm on the right track. I'm moving in the right direction."

The best way to incorporate positive self-talk into your life is to do it every day. In the morning when you wake up, visualize what you want to achieve that day. Write your goals down and read them throughout the day. At night review the goals that you've accomplished and reaffirm your commitment.

Here is an example of a positive self-talk script:

I'm on the right track! I've exercised regularly and have no excuses. I'm moving in the right direction. The more I am able to say this to myself, the more my body will believe it and start creating change. I am loving my body because it has given me so much pleasure and happiness. My body is strong and healthy because I am exercising regularly. This is a beginning of a new era for me - for my health, for my body, and for my life.

- We're more likely to choose healthier food when we think about the benefit it will give us.

Broccoli isn't the tastiest vegetable in the world. In fact, it is rather bitter and boring. But when something might be good for us, we start to see it in a different light. When we think about how healthy it is, how it can lower our cholesterol, how it can prevent cancer or how it is a key component of a healthy diet, it suddenly becomes tastier. That potassium in asparagus, the fiber in beets and the antioxidants in leeks all become a lot more appealing when they are not just delicious, but also good for us.

We all have our favorite foods, or the ones that we crave when we are stressed. So how can we turn those into healthy choices? When we think about the benefits that eating a certain food WON'T bring us, suddenly it becomes much less appealing. Fried chicken is delicious, but it is packed full of fat. Cheese balls are incredibly tasty, but they don't put a dent in our hunger and don't keep us full for long.

The next time you're tempted to choose fried chicken over grilled chicken or potato chips over whole potatoes, think about the things that those foods won't bring you. Think of how hard you'll have to work out at the gym after those indulgences, or how bad the guilt will be when you overeat. The more we think about the negative aspects of a food, the more we won't want it. Being good to ourselves means being mindful of what good things we can eat and how they can help us reach our goals.

**Physiological factors that lead to weight gain**

While it's obvious that we gain weight when we consume more calories than we need, there are other factors that also contribute to our weight gain. The following physiological factors are some of the most common contributors to weight gain.

1. Stress -

Stress is difficult to define and difficult to measure, but it can be measured at the molecular level. The changes in body chemistry after a stressful event can be measured by measuring cortisol, a hormone that is produced during stress and controls several bodily functions including metabolism, growth hormone secretion, immunity, and appetite control. When we release more of this hormone than usual our bodies become stressed with that extra load of cortisol being carried around by the blood for a few days or weeks after the event has passed.

When we're stressed, our appetite increases, we store more fat and are less efficient at using our energy. This can make us gain weight or even become obese.

2. Depression -

Low mood, depression and anxiety all have negative effects on our body's ability to function normally. The higher the severity of these emotions and the longer they go on, the greater the effect they have on weight control. One study showed that when you combine high stress with a lack of sleep, there's an increased chance that you'll gain weight or lose a significant amount of muscle mass because your muscles are not getting any stimulus from hormone release and their ability to use glucose is being impaired.

3. Eating to cope -

Eating is one way that we're able to temporarily relieve stress and take a break from our everyday life. We tend to overeat when we eat for emotional reasons, especially if the food is especially tasty or something we don't get very often (such as pizza or a bag of chips). Weight gain is inevitable when we eat to cope with stress or to simply "comfort eat".

4. Adopting unhealthy habits -

13

Night snacking, eating too quickly, drinking alcohol and not getting enough sleep: All of these things can make it hard to lose weight and can contribute to obesity. It's not so much the loss of calories that we're concerned with when we adopt these habits, but rather the fact that they interfere with our body's ability to burn off calories and process food properly. Metabolism is the process our body uses to burn calories and fat, which is affected by hormones, sleep, exercise and so on.

## Is your mind making you fat?

Mind over matter is an expression that has been used for a long time to describe the idea that our thoughts and emotions can influence our body's physical state. More often than not, it seems to be true. Our mental state can have a major influence on our body's ability to lose weight and have control over their blood sugar levels. Emotions like stress and depression can affect our body's ability to process glucose, which can lead to weight gain and type II diabetes. But how does this hold true in the realm of weight loss? Is there a way of knowing whether our mental state is helping or hindering the weight loss process? Here are five signs that your mindset is holding you back.

A.) You're too ambitious

If you can't break your journey down into discrete chunks, it becomes harder to achieve your goal. Realistic goals are the key to success. Think about setting yourself up for success by breaking big goals into smaller achievable sub-goals. If your goal is to run a marathon, split the task into bite-sized chunks... set a goal to run three miles this week, then build on it from there. It's much easier to successfully reach running five miles than a year later you are still trying to run that first mile.

Can you realistically lose thirty pounds in a month? How are you going to do it? You can't. You will inevitably fail, then feel bad about yourself and perhaps start looking for an easy way out. You may find that you get discouraged, start blaming yourself, and obsessing over the pain you are feeling.

B.) You're not patient.

Losing weight is a process that takes time. Success is a series of failures, repeated in different ways. The key to losing weight is keeping your eye on the bigger picture and not be sidetracked by daily distractions and problems along the way. It's important to keep your long-term goals in mind and be conscious of how challenging it may seem at times, but keep calm, take a deep breath and stick with it! The rewards will come!

It will take at least three months for you to decipher what works for your body. So, give yourself a bit of time, and strive for gradual improvements over a consistent period of time. If you try to do too much too soon, you are setting yourself up for failure. If you think about your weight loss goal as a small baby that needs nurturing and care, you are more likely to succeed than if you treat it like another one of your New Year's resolutions that could easily be forgotten at the stroke of midnight on January 1st.

C. You're not consistent.

It is about the process, not the results. Consistency is key in losing weight and maintaining your results. Everyone is different so there's no definite time period for what we should do to lose weight, but there are some general guidelines that can help you make progress toward your goals: Be consistent – work out three times a week.

15

Be persistent – if you go more than a couple of days without exercising, it's easy to get lazy and give up on your routine. That's why it's important to schedule time on your calendar every week.

### D.) You're not confident about your ability to succeed

If you don't believe that you can make the change or reach your goal, then it's going to be really hard for you to make the changes needed or follow through until you achieve the weight loss results that you want. If you don't think that you can move forward, you will be subconsciously sabotaging yourself.

If you are going to be successful in your weight loss journey, then you must have the necessary confidence to make the necessary changes in your life. Know what steps you need to take to reach your goal. Envision yourself succeeding and making those changes with confidence.

### E.) You're afraid of failure

Putting off change, trying things in a half-hearted manner, or just not trying to change are all behaviors that indicate that you are more comfortable with the status quo. When this happens, you will revert back to the behaviors that were more familiar and more comfortable in the past. When your behavior is reactionary and excuses you from taking action on your own behalf, it's harder to stay committed to making the changes that you know are necessary. When you fear that you'll be judged or ridiculed for making the changes that you need to make, it becomes easier to rely on your current behaviors rather than attempt to change them.

**Changing how we view food**

We can make a mindset shift by changing how we view food. A lack of self-control can be the result of an inability to anticipate the consequences of our actions and follow through with an appropriate response. When you are able to get past the immediate "taste" of a food and imagine yourself after you've eaten it, you are more likely to make an appropriate choice. In other words, if you visualize what it will feel like after you eat too much or after eating something that is less healthy for your body than it is, then that can be a helpful tool in making changes in your mindset. Here are a few introspective questions that can help you to shift that mindset:

- Let's start with one on awareness:

I feel like I should buy a donut. Before I eat one, how many calories does it have Why do I crave one? If I eat it, how long will I need to work out at the gym to burn off these calories? How will eating this donut make me feel in the long-term?

- A question on resilience:

I'm eating a donut and I feel like I'm missing out. How long have I been feeling this way? Is this feeling temporary, or will I still regret eating this donut after an hour? Is the feeling worth eating the donut? How will my body feel like after over-indulging in food and not exercising for a few days, weeks or months? How will my mood be like then? What is the cumulative effect of these choices on my health over time?

- On Responsibility:

If I eat that donut, am I willing to take responsibility for how it will negatively affect every aspect of my life? Will I regret eating it? If I eat a donut, will it make me feel like a failure? Will eating a donut make me feel like a weak person who can't control my eating?

- Here's another one on self-respect:

If I eat this donut, how will it make me feel about myself afterwards? What kind of person makes excuses to eat something that is unhealthy for their body and their mind? Am I proud of the way I am treating myself when I eat junk food or drink alcohol in excess? Do these choices make me feel like a better person or make it?

The goal of these questions is to make you more aware of how your current choices affect your life, the lives of those around you, and ultimately the world. This awareness can help you reshape your unhealthy behaviors into choices that are healthier for your mind, body and spirit.

There are many ways to make any sort of change in life, but with a little consistent effort and some introspection, it's possible to become more disciplined so that you can live a healthier life. Get into the habit of buying at least one healthy food every time you go grocery shopping with the goal being to gradually adding more healthy foods to your diet. Keep a food journal and update it every time you eat unhealthy foods so that you can see how much progress you're making.

- Food for thought:

Revisiting the moments in life when limiting beliefs held you back.

As we end this chapter, I want you to revisit some of the moments in your life when limiting beliefs were holding you back. Maybe there was that time you were too scared to ask out that person you liked. Perhaps you wanted to apply for a job, but you were too nervous to go in for an interview. Or maybe you felt like you weren't good enough to get into that college, so you settled for second-best.

Consider all the missed opportunities, friendships, and relationships that you could have built over the years if your limiting beliefs did not keep getting in the way.

The goal of this exercise isn't to feel bad about yourself. No one can change the past, but what you can do is learn from your past mistakes so that you don't repeat them.

This exercise is also meant to give you an opportunity to reframe the negative thoughts and beliefs that have been holding you back. You now have the knowledge and the tools to work towards building a life that feels right for you. It's time to put your past behind you and start getting excited about your future. Limiting beliefs don't just hold us back from meeting our fitness goals, they also keep us from living a purposeful life.

In the next chapter, we'll be looking at how we can change what we think about weight loss and how we can be more accepting and forgiving of ourselves.

# CHAPTER 2

# The beliefs that weigh us down

**How the fitness industry makes us buy stuff we don't need**

Upto 67% of gym memberships go unused. Can we blame ourselves? Maybe. The fitness industry has made it too easy for us to get a dopamine rush by acquiring new workout equipment and gym clothes. The advent of social media and online selling, makes it too easy for us to be influenced by messages from friends and society at large. Most people have a hard time rejecting things that we see as attractive. We make commitments that we don't follow up on, because after all, our minds are easily swayed when it comes to making decisions about what we want.

We are also at the mercy of marketers when it comes to food. A large portion of our food budget goes towards junk foods and sugary drinks that we don't need much. And let's face it, marketing is pretty effective when it comes to selling us things like fast food and processed junk.

It's no wonder that some people decide to become gym members once they join the workforce or get married. They have no idea how much time they'll actually spend at the gym and they're scared of missing out on friends and networking opportunities because of their lack of physical fitness and social skills.

The weight loss industry is a multi-billion-dollar industry. Why? Because they've mastered the art of using marketing and the human mind to trick people into buying things that they don't really need. Diet pills that don't work, creams that can't help you lose weight, and diet plans that are too extreme. These gimmicky products look legit and while some of them might work, they don't last. Sure, you lose a few pounds, but it's not sustainable. The creators of these products are not so much interested in helping you lose weight as they are in getting your money. Like Bernie Madoff in the finance industry, weight loss product creators have built a system that's too enticing for people to resist and now the weight loss industry is losing its credibility because the general feeling is that most diet plans and supplements don't work.

**Some of the lies we've been fed**

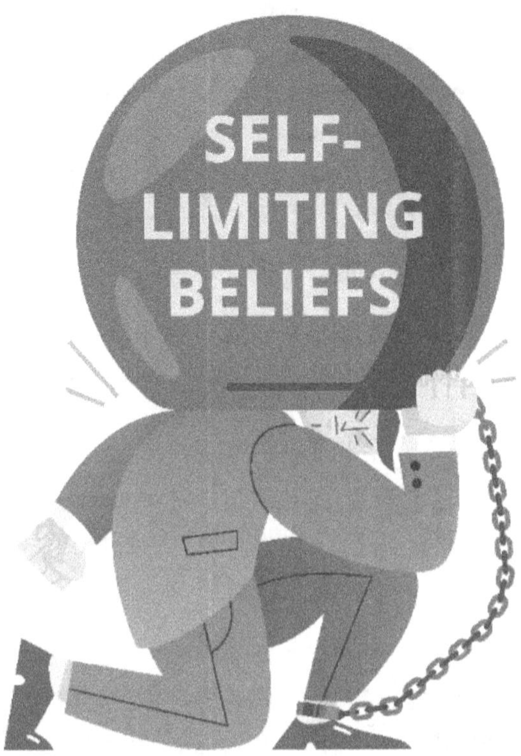


Marketers are partly to blame for feeding us with lies and half-truths that are intended to persuade us to believe in the products. Sometimes these beliefs aren't spread with malicious but just that they don't provide us with enough information to form an informed opinion. Here are some common harmful weight loss beliefs and how these can also be applied to healthy living.


**1. We should avoid certain food groups**

In weight loss circles, carbs or fats are demonized. You always hear that carbs are fattening, and that eating fat is bad for the heart. But a calorie is a calorie – the burning of food in our body does not depend on what type of carbohydrate or fat it is. So should you avoid them to lose weight? Of course not! Carbs and fats are an important source of energy for our bodies. They give us endurance, help us maintain our mood and help us feel full after we eat something small. But having too much of these types of foods can also be a problem because they're more likely to make you overeat later on in the day – so their bad side will eventually catch up with you.

This belief is dangerous because it encourages us to avoid many healthy foods that we should eat such as whole grains, beans and root vegetables. It's no surprise then that a diet that is low in carbs and fat tends to be higher in refined sugars and trans fats. The solution is to cut down on the amount of refined carbohydrates you eat while adding more healthy carbs (whole grains) to your diet.

Instead of saying that carbs are bad, the solution is to focus on the quality of carbs you're eating so you can maximize their benefits and minimize their drawbacks. When you eat a cup of whole grain cereal which is high in fiber and complex carbs, you get the biggest benefit from eating it.

## 2. All calories are equal

This is the opposite of the first belief. While it's true that all calories are not created equal – some are more easily used by the body than others, and some have no nutritional value at all! Some foods can also be digested more slowly by your body resulting in a slower absorption of energy. This means you'll be less likely to overeat later on in the day.

When the "calories in = calories out" weight loss model is used extensively without acknowledgment of the different types of calories, it can be misleading. It's impossible to understand how the body works without acknowledging the different effects that different foods and drinks have on your body.

For example, protein, vegetables, and fruit are easily and quickly digested by your body but they don't provide you with a lot of energy. On the other hand, fats are slow to digest and can also be used by your body as energy, especially when you're working out since they're more readily available as fuel.

Foods that have fiber can be useful in weight loss because they make you feel fuller for longer even if their calorie content may not be that high. Foods may have the same number of calories, but they can have very different effects on your body – depending on their type and how much you eat them. The insulin response and metabolic effects are also different with some foods and drinks.

Reducing the amount of fat in your diet (while still eating the right amount of protein) can also help you lose weight because it's easier for your body to burn fat for energy than it is to break down carbohydrates. Rather than focusing solely on cutting carbs, focus on how much fat you eat, how often you eat them and what type of fats you're consuming.

**3. We need to starve ourselves to lose weight**

25

Although it's true that not eating anything for a few hours can make you lose weight, most people don't realize this. They're also not aware of how harmful this habit is to their health. Losing weight can be achieved through healthy eating and regular exercise. People who've gone on crash diets have been found to be more prone to serious illnesses and even death because they're starving themselves.

To live healthy, a balance needs to be reached between your overall calorie intake and your activity levels. You should eat food that will keep you full throughout the day while still being relatively low in calories so you can control your hunger and eat less than you need each day.

Extreme modifications of intermittent fasting can be unhealthy if you do it for too long and if you're not eating properly. Instead, try to find a healthy balance between your diet and exercise.

When we starve ourselves, our bodies go into survival mode. To save energy and to prevent muscle loss, our bodies slow down the metabolism. This is all good if you're in a life-or-death situation but not when it comes to losing weight. When this happens, your body will hold on to fat even if you're exercising regularly. When it does, the body will convert your muscle into energy instead of using the body fat in an effort to slow down your metabolism.

**4. We need to lose weight to be attractive/loved/happy**

There's a lot of pressure to look good and be skinny nowadays. Many women are insecure about their bodies because the media portrays only the young and fit as attractive. Since it's impossible for most people to become exactly like that, many suffer from eating disorders or depression.

There is nothing wrong with wanting to improve yourself. But we need to understand that if we focus too much on our looks or weight, we may be overlooking other important qualities – such as character, intelligence, or humor. If your weight loss methods make you thinner but you feel worse inside, then they're not working.

When fashion magazines are used to making people feel insecure about their bodies, we need to realize that they're more fiction than truth. If you're not happy with the way you look, then you'll still be unhappy no matter how much weight you lose.

A positive self-image is the result of a healthy body, not the other way around. Don't lose yourself trying to be something you're not! Instead, work on your inner self and love yourself for who you are now. It's perfectly fine if you don't look like a model. You can still be both fit and fine without constantly worrying about your weight and how others see you.

## 5. We should be ashamed of being overweight/obese

Fat shaming is an intolerant idea that needs to be stopped. We shouldn't have to live in a world where people are judged based on their looks and weight. Making fun of someone for being overweight is no different than making fun of someone because of their race or religion.

27

Being obese means, you're facing some health issues (such as diabetes) which can reduce your quality of life, but it doesn't make you any less human than anyone else. We shouldn't be ashamed or embarrassed to be overweight; we should embrace our bodies and accept who we are while working hard to improve ourselves through healthy eating and exercise.

This false belief that obesity is a character flaw, rather than a health issue, also leads to people treating and shaming each other based on weight. Often this can lead to bullying against overweight people.

If we are going to have a dialogue about obesity, then let's talk about it in a mature and productive manner. There's a way to overcome feelings of shame and learn to love your body. Our self-esteem shouldn't be linked to our weight but to how we feel about ourselves and how comfortable we are with who we are.

## 6. There's an "ideal" body shape

The apple, the pear, the triangle, and the other geometric shapes that we have created to describe body shapes are not realistic. If you've ever looked at the "ideal" shape on a magazine cover, then you already know that it's completely unattainable for most (or all) women.

There are many different types of body shapes. While some are just naturally slenderer than others – some people may be overweight due to genetics or other factors that can't be changed. Instead of thinking about how we could change our bodies to look like the "ideal" one, we should focus on what we can do to have a healthier lifestyle and accept our bodies for who and what they are.

There's a difference between setting your standards and having unrealistic expectations. Not setting any standards at all is also unhealthy. If we want to be healthier, then we need to work towards our goals while accepting ourselves along the way.

We should focus on our health rather than what we look like naked. But at the same time, our body image should be more than just a reflection of what we see in a mirror. We need to have confidence in who we are and how much value we add to other people's lives in order for us to be happy and healthy.

**Why the scale is flawed**

A bathroom scale is an important part of our everyday life. We rely on it to keep track of how much we eat and to track our weight throughout the day. But weighing yourself is not something that you need to do every day. In fact, it can be demotivating if done too frequently. But why is it that we do this more than once every day? It must be because we're psyched about the number that the scale shows, isn't it?

Maybe this is just a harmless habit or maybe there's more to it. Here are a few reasons why you shouldn't weigh yourself often:

**You'll obsess over your weight**

When you're relying on a scale to tell you how much you weigh each day, then you'll be obsessing over losing weight as well. If the number goes up, then that means you've gained weight, and vice versa if it goes down. It makes sense if done only once a week but not if done daily. When done too often, weighing yourself will affect your mood and self-esteem based on one single number. Instead of getting obsessed with the number that appears on the scale, you should focus on how your clothes are fitting or how your body is changing.

The number on the scale doesn't tell you everything. Your weight is not the only factor in determining your health and fitness. Muscle weighs more than fat so you may be heavier but not necessarily unhealthy. You may have gained weight but it's still possible that it's muscle rather than fat if you've been exercising regularly. You might be losing fat or gaining muscle depending on your workout and diet.

**Weight fluctuations are a thing**

Fluid retention, constipation, current glycogen levels, water retention, metabolic rate, temperature, and stress are all factors that can affect your weight fluctuations. When you weigh yourself too often, then you won't get to see how much of an effect those factors have on your weight.

Body composition is a great way to track your progress in terms of fat loss or muscle gain. The scale is not meant for this purpose as it only measures how much total weight there is on the body. In order to see how much fat or muscle you actually have, you need to buy a body composition scale and measure your waist, hips, and arms with a tape measure while wearing the same clothes that you wore before the weigh-in.

## You might be underestimating your weight loss

If you weigh yourself often, then you may be underestimating the amount of weight that you're losing. So, for example, if you weigh yourself every morning and find out that yesterday was a good day to lose weight (because the number went down), then that means it's normal for the number to go down on a bad day or even on a good day when you're not trying to lose weight. The way your body reacts to the pounds lost or gained is unique. You'll never know what causes the difference unless you track your weight yourself.

## The scale is a feedback mechanism, not a tool to judge yourself by

When you weigh yourself, then it's only a way to see how your diet and exercise have affected your body throughout the day. It can give you useful info about how much fat or muscle you've gained or lost but it shouldn't be used as a tool to judge yourself. The scale shouldn't be a way for you to feel shame if it goes up. You shouldn't feel better about yourself if the number goes down either. Use it as a tool to track your progress but never as a tool to measure your self-worth.

## Rethinking weight loss

The terms "weight loss" and "fat loss" are used interchangeably, leading many to think that the two mean the same thing. Of course, fat loss is the largest factor in weight loss.

But weight is just a measure of mass. It doesn't tell you how much fat you have on your body or how much muscle you have. And it doesn't tell you the health status of your body. I've talked about this before when we looked at why the scale shouldn't be your only measuring stick. If you want to know what your body looks like, the best way to do it is by having a look at yourself in the mirror. When we lose fat without seeing a drop on the scale, it's usually because we've lost fat and replaced it with muscle.

Rethinking weight loss starts with changing our mindset. Instead of obsessing over numbers, start looking at how you feel. Our energy levels, mood, skin, hair. etc. Rethinking weight loss means that we do away with a one size fits all approach to dieting. In order for this to happen, we have to stop using the word diet. Diet implies that our bodies are temporary and that they need to be changed or manipulated until they look a certain way. When it comes down to it, what makes us healthy isn't our body size or numbers on a scale; it's how well we treat our bodies every day. And treating yourself well isn't about fitting into pre-determined standards of beauty.

Let's start by looking at how even little changes on the scale can have a big impact on your overall health. What impact does a 3-pound weight loss have? A 5% reduction in body weight is enough to reduce the risk of diabetes, heart disease and some cancers. And by losing 10 percent of your body weight, you can reduce your risk of developing osteoarthritis, sleep apnea and improve many aspects of your cardiovascular health. Aside from that, it's motivating when we realize that it doesn't take a huge lifestyle change to see progress. Successful weight loss doesn't have to mean completely altering your lifestyle. It can be as simple as making good food choices and getting in a few extra steps every day.

Instead of aiming for that glorious transformation where you envision yourself with a flat tummy and toned thighs, ask yourself what success would look like to you. How will you know if you're on the right track? A great way to set a goal is by focusing on process rather than results. In other words, think about what you have to do to achieve your goal.

Having a healthy body doesn't mean you have to be thin. It's no secret that there is a social pressure to have a certain body type in this country. But there are so many other factors that determine our health and well-being than just the number on a scale. Feeling your best is also about being more active, getting more sleep, and being less stressed out by food rules and restrictions.

**Tracking the things that matter**

Your weight isn't the only thing that matters here. You want to see what your body is made up of. What are you losing and gaining? So, don't worry about the scale, forget about those numbers and start tracking how you feel. Are you more motivated? Do you have more energy? Are you sleeping better? If so, then keep doing what you're doing. Keep up the good work! If not, then it's time to make some changes.

Keeping track of how you feel is a good way to keep you motivated. Even when things get a little tough, it's easy to take a step back and ask yourself what possible reward is worth the sacrifice. It's much less overwhelming than seeing numbers on a scale go down and then trying to figure out why the number went up.

It's important that we don't focus too much on losing weight or gaining weight but rather focus on healthy eating and getting as much activity as we can. The end goal is to lose weight, the journey is the important part.

So, get tracking! Keep a food journal, take your measurements, and record how you sleep. Keep track of all the things that matter most to you, aside from the scale, and see how it affects your overall health. It doesn't matter if the number goes up, if you're feeling great then keep doing what you're doing. You can always use the scale to measure progress over time but don't try to tell yourself that weighing yourself is a measure of self-worth or that it defines who you are as a person.

The ideal weight isn't one where you are magically skinny, or a given number on a scale. It's when your body looks and feels healthy, whether that's through a little extra muscle, a little less fat, or even the same weight as you used to be. Whether it takes a few extra pounds to reach that goal isn't important. In fact, working towards that goal can be much more rewarding than the end result. Rethinking weight loss is an attitude adjustment and refocusing on things that actually matter, like energy levels, mood, appearance, or how you feel in your clothes. Now that all seems much more important than the number on the scale!

**A mindful approach to dieting and weight loss**

Instead of viewing your body as a temporary thing that needs to be changed, start viewing it as the home of your health. Treating yourself well isn't only about exercise and clean eating; it's also about getting enough sleep, staying stress free, giving yourself some time to relax and finding ways to cheer up or calm down when you're stressed out or anxious. As we get older, we realize that drastic changes in our lives aren't as easy as they once were. We realize that making any big changes can be extremely stressful and anxiety-provoking. A lifestyle change like dieting is no exception. It just becomes a whole lot easier to do when your body is feeling well, your mind is clear, and you're not caught up in food rules and restrictions. So, when you start to feel those feelings of pressure or stress about weight loss, remember that the purpose of the journey isn't the end goal but rather the process. The process of healthy eating, getting enough exercise every day and treating yourself well so that you can continue to stay healthy for years to come. Here are a few things that will help you view weight loss (and wellness in general) in a way that makes you feel more confident and less stressed.

### Forget about obsessively counting calories.

It's all about paying attention to yourself and your daily diet. Consuming fewer calories than you burn up is a surefire way to weight loss and the best way to gain muscle and lose fat at the same time. You don't need to track every single calorie, but you do need to have an idea of what you're eating. Obsessive calorie counting takes the fun out of eating. We're mammals and being surrounded by delicious food is a positive thing. It's necessary to remember that eating should be fun and that it should be rewarding. In fact, being in the kitchen and prepping healthy meals should be a point of pride. A lifestyle change like dieting shouldn't be something that takes away from your quality of life.

### Dieting isn't a punishment.

Instead of viewing dieting as a punishment and a way to punish yourself, you can view it instead as a learning experience. It's how you get to know yourself better. You learn how your body works, what it likes and dislikes and how to cook more healthy meals for yourself. You learn what works for your body and what doesn't. You also learn about foods that will make you feel good about yourself. By changing the foods that you eat, we become more mindful of our actions and are much less likely to overeat when we're in the mood for something unhealthy.

When you say that you won't get that ice cream, you're not "punishing" yourself. You're giving your body the nutrients and vitamins it needs. You are not a bad or unworthy person if you slip up and have ice cream every once in a while.

## Food isn't a reward either

Food is fuel. You don't need a reason to eat those yummy cookies. Don't say "I can't have a cookie" instead substitute it with "I don't need a cookie" or even better, "I don't want a cookie." That's not to say that you can't have a cookie sometimes, in fact, it's important that you realize that it's OK to treat yourself sometimes. Rewarding yourself for weight loss is one thing but if you think of food as a reward then you start to associate all of your self-worth with the stuff you eat. It also makes it seem like eating food is more exciting than doing other activities and may lead to overindulgence. Sure, ice cream tastes much better after a nice long walk through the park but you don't need to eat it to make yourself feel better.

## There are no "good" or "bad" foods

This black-and-white thinking is a trap that we fall into regularly. Foods are not good or bad – they are just foods. They can be enjoyed and even loved, but one puny thing shouldn't completely invalidate a food as a whole. The more you think about it, the more you'll realize that this is true- except for maybe poison ivy, that stuff is bad news.

You'll also notice how you get enthralled by the idea of "bad" foods sometimes. "But cheese tastes so good", or "I just love ice cream". To think of those foods as the demon spawns of Satan is silly and doesn't really help us figure out how to manage them better. We only end up beating ourselves up and feeling bad because we ate them. Instead of demonizing food, think of them as a little bonus to help you avoid that extra 500 calories. You don't need the food to feel good or to be healthy. Even if you eat something that you know is bad for you, it doesn't mean that you're worthless because you ate it, and it doesn't mean that your weight loss hasn't been successful. A journey towards wellness and weight loss doesn't have to be painful. It can be exciting and fun!

**Is that weight loss plan sustainable?**

For a weight loss strategy to be sustainable, which means that it will work in the long term, it must meet these three basic criteria in order to be considered.

**1.) It must work for you**

The plan must take into accord your individual needs, and it must work for your lifestyle. If you find yourself constantly feeling frustrated or restricted, or if the foods on your plan don't appeal to you, then it's not sustainable. You may burnout on that plan and blame your body, food and weight for your inability to

37

stick to a diet. You may feel like nothing you are doing is working. Everything you see points to a failure of some sort, which will cause you to dig into feel down and depressed.

## 2.) It must be easy to maintain

Your plan must be easy to maintain, which means that you're able to fit your healthy eating plan into your daily life. It also means that you should be able to stick with it without major challenges for the rest of your life. Willpower is a limited resource, and if you're constantly falling short, you're going to exhaust your willpower and you'll end up giving in to temptation. You won't be able to maintain the process or stay on track day after day.

## 3.) It must be realistic

Not only must your plan be sustainable, but it must also be realistic. Will you still be able to follow your plan when you're at a party with friends? Can you stick with your plan while traveling or during a stressful period at work? If you're on the verge of quitting, then it's not something that is realistic for your lifestyle.

What will happen when you fall off the wagon? Take a second to think about what you're going to do when you fall off the wagon. Most people who lose weight and then gain it all back don't look at what they'll do when they take a fall. Will you go and eat a carton of ice cream or cookies out of depression? Will you go for one week or two weeks and say "Hey, I failed, I might as well give up now?" What happens when life gets busy, your schedule changes, or you decide that this isn't worth the effort anymore? You need to have a contingency plan ready.

## Noticing progress

We saw that the scale is only one of the numerous ways of measuring how you're doing in your weight loss journey. There are many other ways to measure body changes that you can see. Knowing what to look for can help you know if your weight loss plan is working or if it needs to be tweaked a little.

> ### A shrinking waist size

When clothes fit differently, it's an early indicator of weight change. Old clothes will start to fit looser, and new clothes that you buy will fit better. This is an easy thing to measure without a scale.

> ### New muscle definition

You can look for definition in your biceps, your inner thighs, your forearms and in the back of your upper arms. Being able to see these little muscles under the fat is a good sign that you're working with what you have and not against it.

> ### Lower blood pressure

Blood pressure can be measured at home using a blood pressure monitor or sometimes just by checking it at the doctor's office. The heart will no longer strain to pump as much blood around your body because it doesn't have to travel through fat tissue. The blood pressure will lower, leaving you with a nice energy boost.

> ### Increased energy levels

As your body begins to function better, you'll notice an increase in energy levels. You won't feel so bloated and uncomfortable all the time. You won't be dragging yourself around feeling lethargic after every meal because your body isn't working against itself anymore. Instead of feeling like there's a big, lead ball in your chest, you'll have more energy and be able to think clearer.

> **A loss in inches**

This is one of the most important things to keep an eye out for. As you lose weight, your body will begin to shape up and you'll notice that you no longer have a spare tire around your middle. The skin will begin to tighten, and that spare tire will start to disappear. If you are trying a crash diet, then this is not something that you should be expecting. It can take weeks or months for this change to happen.

**Food for thought: Writing down your weight loss milestones**

In this chapter, we've seen that a weight loss plan is not just a series of diet rules and restrictions. It should be a detailed strategy that takes into account your needs, your lifestyle, and the results that you want to see. It should help you lose weight and keep it off for the long term.

We've seen how the scale isn't necessarily an accurate way to measure your body changes. You can measure changes in other ways such as shrinking waist size, more defined muscles, lower blood pressure levels, increased energy levels and a loss in inches from around your waistline. Keep track of your food intake using tools like MyFitnessPal or an app for your smartphone.

I want you to think about how you can measure your success as you continue your journey towards weight loss. As much as I've encouraged you to set small daily steps in the right direction, they take time to add up. It's important to keep track of these small steps and to celebrate them as much as the big milestones.

You may want to set some healthy eating and exercise goals for yourself. Write them down so you can refer to them at any time. You might want to revisit your goals every six months or so, and make sure that they fit in with where you are now and where you want to be in the future.

Write down your weight loss milestones in your notebook, on your computer, or in some other place where you will see them. You might have to put these milestones on the wall or put them on the refrigerator with a magnet. These are tangible goals that you can use as markers for progress.

These milestones will be in form of a checklist. Here are some examples:

- Lost two sizes in clothes and hosiery. My old clothes feel loose now.

- Can walk on the treadmill for five minutes without feeling breathless.

- I have reached my goal weight and have maintained it for 6 months. I no longer think about food all day long, obsessively counting calories and fat grams.

- Took a photo of myself in my underwear to support my success in losing weight and keeping it off.

- I have increased my energy levels. I feel energized and full of energy every day now.

When you take photos of your progress, document the date and keep it in your notes so you can look back on them when you are happy with your success and amazed at your achievements. Not just for other people to see but also for yourself so that you can see how far you've come and how far you still need to go.

What does success mean to you? What are your goals and milestones? What would you like to achieve? How do you plan on achieving these goals and milestones? Any steps that you'd like to share with us? Write more about this in your journal.

# CHAPTER 3

43

# The magic in thinking positively

We're constantly bombarded with negative news and an over-abundance of negative thoughts, especially news that makes us dwell on how depressing the state of the world is. So, if you've lost a few pounds, or if you do manage to lose weight and keep it off for a while, you're fine one day—and then BAM! You hit a plateau. You're no longer losing weight. You've hit another brick wall. One of the keys to staying motivated and believing in your success when you feel like giving up is to focus on the progress that you have already made rather than focusing on where you are now and what "failure" looks like.

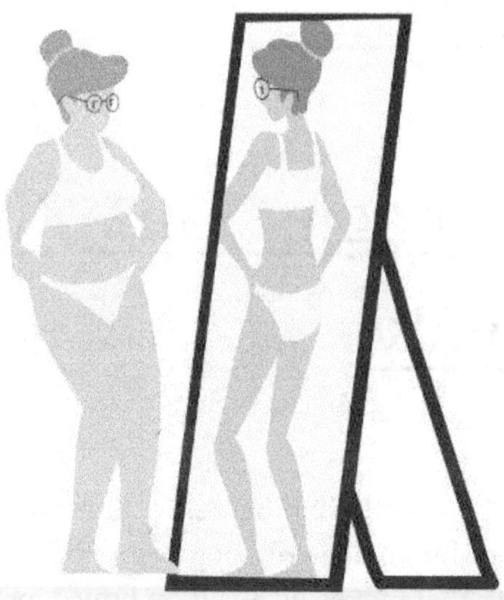

Nutritionists often suggest not to focus on weight loss, but rather to focus on changing your eating habits instead of obsessing about the number on the scale. Weight loss is a side effect of changing your eating habits, rather than focusing on weight loss itself. You need to focus on what you can do, not what can't be done. In a way, our weight is a reflection of our thoughts and our emotions.

Let's examine another very common scenario. You've been counting calories and you've cut way back on fat and sugar, which are often the culprits when it comes to weight gain. You're eating six small meals a day, eating tons of vegetables and fruits, drinking more water, you've joined a gym and you're working out regularly. You really think that all is going well until one day you go to the doctor's office and find out that your cholesterol is a little high.

This isn't what you expected at all! You've been eating healthy and exercising like crazy but still your cholesterol levels are not in the green zone. It doesn't matter if you've been exercising, eating healthy foods and drinking water... Your cholesterol levels are still going up. The reason why you haven't lost any weight or haven't seen any dramatic changes in your waist size is because there is probably a whole other story that goes on inside your body. There are so many things happening back there that the doctors aren't even aware of.

The next day, you go to another doctor for blood work and find out that your triglycerides—an important factor in determining heart health —are a little low. You're not happy but you don't get too worried yet because it might have been just random numbers from random tests from different doctors, different labs, different health centers.

Should you be alarmed when the numbers are low? Not necessarily, because you can have high triglycerides and still be healthy. How we view ourselves and our bodies is a reflection of the diet and lifestyle that we are living. This is why it's so important to look at all the components of our lives and see how they fit together.

A few days later, you go for a full checkup, which includes an EKG, stress test, blood work, urinalysis and more. The doctor tells you that your heart is healthy and there are no signs of any type of disease or infection. They tell you that everything looks great! External statistics, such as your cholesterol and triglycerides, don't tell the whole story. Your internal body image is far more important.

It's the same thing when it comes to losing weight. If you have a healthy weight to start with, you will reach a point where you feel happy with yourself. You'll start experiencing less stress in your daily life and your mind will feel lighter and more at ease. Within this mental state, you'll be much more open to change and new ideas that can positively impact upon your body image, physical health, and overall well-being.

**What are negative thoughts?**

Why are thoughts like: "I'm not thin enough", "I'm too fat", "I need to lose more weight", "My waist size is too large", "I need to work out more", "I should be able to eat a lot more (carbohydrates) or less (fat)?" How can these thoughts prevent you from making positive changes in your life?

When you think negatively, it's very difficult to believe in your own success. You're constantly comparing yourself to others and realizing that they have it easier than you do. The word "easy" is thrown around a lot these days and it makes people feel like they're not doing enough, when really, we all have our own limitations. That's why we have goals and milestones instead.

Are you having a bad day? Why not try to think of something positive? Try to think about the next step and what you want to achieve from this step. Think about your success, how far you've come and how far you still need to go. Try not to just try to change your body weight or waist size, or even see results in one area of your life—try to work on improving all areas of your life simultaneously. This is when positive thinking really kicks in—

when we're not focused on negative thoughts, we start seeing our lives as they are and not as what they're going to be with unrealistic expectations.

## A hole in the ship

How do thoughts hold us back from seeing results? They can be upsetting, depressing and fearful when we look at our weight. Thinking in a way that doesn't work with our body's natural cycles and rhythms can actually make it harder to lose weight.

The following are some of the main ways that negative thinking holds us back and how we can turn things around:

1).Thinking in a very black and white way without considering the grey areas.

When you start dieting, many people think "I need to lose 10 pounds." If they manage to lose 5 pounds, instead of the targeted 10 pounds, they're not as happy and think that they've failed. Negative thoughts like these can cause you to lose confidence and motivation. While 5 pounds is still better than 0 pounds, it's more important to focus on the positive changes we're making.

2.) Difficulty in accepting the truth.

The truth is that it's not all about the number on the scale. A "bad" day at work or a bad night's sleep can affect our mood and our weight. There are many factors that go into a healthy body such as our eating habits, physical activity levels, how much we

47

sleep, and many other things. Dieting doesn't make us lose weight—it's how we live our life that does so.

**3.)** Intrinsic motivation doesn't work in a negative environment.

Intrinsic motivation or doing something because it's fun and makes us happy, is a great motivator. Instead of focusing on how much (or little) weight we've lost in a month, try to focus on the experience and how much fun you're having with your activities. Stay positive by reminding yourself that weight loss is a process—it's not always going to be easy and we're going to have good days and bad days.

**4.)** We sabotage ourselves with negative thoughts.

Many people take on diets as a temporary thing and subconsciously start saying things like "this diet won't last forever" or "I'll be able to eat whatever I want when I reach my goal weight." These types of thoughts can lead to you eating fattening foods and feel guilty about it because you've already given yourself permission to eat anything once you lose the weight. Thoughts like this assume that this lifestyle change is a temporary one and that something will make you gain the weight back.

**5.)** Undermining Self-Esteem.

It's important to have a good sense of self-esteem and self-worth, but it doesn't help that we continuously tell ourselves that we don't deserve to be happy, healthy, or successful. We can sabotage ourselves through self-doubt and low self-esteem. The more often you hear yourself say this, the more you will believe it. Keep in mind that it takes a lot of energy to maintain negative thoughts. It's not just "thinking" as such; it's "perpetuating" thought patterns that are hardwired into our brain.

**6.)** Emotional Eating.

Emotional eating is when we eat when we are upset, anxious, or stressed out. In the short term, it can be a quick fix to make us feel better, but in the long term it's not healthy; in fact, it can make things much worse. The more you think negatively, the more likely you are to be drawn towards food as a source of comfort and as a result causing you to gain weight.

**7.)** Comparing Yourself to Others

It's okay if you don't look like the models you see in magazines, but when you think that all of your friends are having fun and enjoying themselves, while you're stuck at home doing nothing and feeling miserable all the time; it's not healthy. Everyone is going through different things in their lives and everyone thinks about food differently, so don't compare yourself to other people—compare yourself to your own previous performance.

**Cultivating positive thinking**

It's only natural that we feel down when we've had a rough day, or our life is in shambles. But if we get stuck in that funk for too long, we can't lose excess weight. We all live in our own reality. That's why a positive attitude is so important not just for losing weight but for just about everything. You need to have positive thoughts, or you'll feel overwhelmed by all the negativity around you. When you're in a good mood, it's easier to make good

49

choices. Here are some ways you can boost your mood and jumpstart your weight loss:

> **Start a weight loss journal.**

Life is full of ups and downs, but it's the downs that you need to pay attention to. In times of stress, writing things down helps you to stay on top of things. It also helps you to see the big picture. Be sure to write down what you ate and how your weight is changing in your journal. When you look back on these entries a couple of months from now, isn't it comforting to see that the upward trend was temporary and that your weight loss still continues? Journalling is also a simple and effective way to boost your mood. Sometimes you just need to get things off your chest, and writing is a great release.

> **Adopt SMART weight loss goals**

Simple goals are also realistic, and they're easier to achieve. If your goal is too big, you might get discouraged after a couple of setbacks and give up. If you break it down into smaller steps, it becomes much more manageable. Let's say your ultimate goal is to lose 50 lbs. If that seems like an impossible feat right now, break it down into smaller goals like losing 5 lbs in a month; losing 10 lbs. in two months; and so on. Break the process into the smallest possible steps so that you can enjoy each victory along the way!

Smart goals are Specific, Measurable, Attainable, Realistic, and Time-bound. Specific means that your goal is clear, detailed, and written down in a place where you can easily access it. Measurable means that you can quantify your goal. You can measure the distance you've walked in a day, the number of times you've been in the gym, or how much water you've consumed.

Attainable means that you know that you can accomplish it. A goal is achievable when it is within your control, and it's not affected by outside influences. Realistic means that your goal aligns with your overall vision, and it is something that you can actually do. Time-bound makes deadlines for achieving your goals.

> **Visualize the end goal.**

After you make your goal, write it down, rehearse or visualize yourself achieving it. This will keep your subconscious in check and will help you to do everything in your power to reach that goal. Get excited about the end result. Think about how good it will make you feel when you've reached that target weight. Picture yourself fitting into those smaller clothes and looking great at your next big event! This might seem unrelated, but did you know that there is a strong connection between the mind and body? By feeding yourself positive thoughts and powerful images, we are training our minds to perform the tasks necessary for success. How different will your life be after you've reached that target weight? What kinds of things will you do? How will your self-confidence grow after attaining your goal? These are the questions you want to be asking yourself. You'll be surprised how good it makes you feel to accomplish a goal – even if it's a small one. Have a way to deal with negative emotions.

Negative emotions can also lead to a weight loss plateau. When you're in a rut, it's hard to motivate yourself to work out or even look at your diet plan. Staying positive and focusing on the good things in your life will help you beat this hurdle. When you feel down, think of the best thing that happened to you that day or how proud you are of a person who is close to you. If you can't find something good, think of the one thing you can do to make yourself feel better. Think of a time when you've achieved major milestones in your life like graduating from high school or starting university or getting into a great new job. These are just some examples: how about making it through your finals? Or getting that promotion? A new job? Getting married? Thinking about these things will help get you out of your funk.

Going for a small walk when you don't feel like it will also help boost your mood. You'll be surprised at how much better you'll feel after doing a couple of minutes of regular exercise. It will also help you to reach a healthy weight and keep it there. Walking is considered a low-impact form of exercise, so it won't put too much stress on your joints. Plus, the more you do it, the better you'll get at finding your rhythm and enjoy it more and more as time goes on.

> **Find new friends who push you to do more.**

We're social creatures, so we all want to feel like part of the group. When you meet new people, look for those who will support and encourage you on your weight loss journey. Try to avoid negative people who will bring you down. If someone is always putting others down, spoiling your mood and making light of your goals, don't spend time with them. You deserve better! If possible, join a weight-loss support group where you can share your struggles and successes with others who are in the same boat as you. Talking to others who are in the same position as you is a great way to stay accountable and be motivated by them as well.

Your local gym might also have weight loss support groups or weight watchers' meetings. I've been going to my gym's monthly meetings for a few months now, and it helps to listen to others share their experiences and learn from them. It's also a good way for me to check in with myself and make sure that I'm staying on track with my diet and exercise.

## How do you Sustain Positive Thinking?

Adopting a positive thinking approach will help you to reach your health goals. After you've set up a system that works for you, stick with it! You can still have fun and enjoy life while you're losing weight. You'll find that the more you focus on your health, the easier it is to reach your goals. It will be a more enjoyable process and chances are, you'll look forward to doing something good for yourself. Keep in mind that your attitude is a powerful tool that you have in your control. If you think positively, chances are you'll get positive results. By staying positive and feeding yourself positive thoughts, images, and actions, you can make your goals a reality. Staying on the path will be easier with these things.

## 1. Don't give up when you slip up

When you think about reaching your goals and you start to feel discouraged, remember that you're doing something good for yourself. You're giving yourself the gift of looking as good as possible. A setback can be an opportunity to learn more about yourself and how to set up your healthy eating plan more effectively. You will fall off the track a few times before you find your stride. That is totally normal! If you don't give up, you will lose weight and be able to keep it off. Setbacks are opportunities to learn more about yourself, adjust your strategy, and use your lessons learned in the future to make more successful decisions.

Realize that mistakes are a part of life. Even people who do everything right sometimes slip up and indulge in foods they shouldn't eat. Life happens, as they say! When you make a mistake, forgive yourself, learn from it – especially if you haven't done it many times before – and try again.

See the lesson in learning to accept your mistakes, forgive yourself and try again. Don't use it as a way to justify giving up on your goals. Forgive yourself and move on!

Sometimes we do things out of a place of sadness or insecurity and that is never an excuse to eat poorly or skip exercise. If you do find yourself making poor decisions out of a state of sadness, you can always turn to a good friend for help or see if there's something in your life that you can change to make you feel happier.

## 2. Ditch perfectionism.

I know how hard it can be, but if you can, try to let go of the idea that you have to be perfect in order for your weight loss plan to be effective and a success. There is no such thing as the perfect diet and exercise routine. I'm not saying you shouldn't eat healthy and work out – of course you should! What I'm saying is that it's not always possible to do everything perfectly all the time, especially when life gets in the way. If you slip up on your diet or exercise, don't get discouraged and give up. Keep going as best as you can, forgive yourself for your imperfections, learn from them, and move forward with your goals.

Sometimes you need to accept your imperfections and realize that you're just not going to be perfect 100% of the time no matter how hard you try. Sometimes life happens and there's nothing you can do about it. It's important to realize this because feeling guilty about every little thing you do wrong will only make you feel worse, which in turn, makes it even harder for you to stick with your goals.

### 3. Find a support system.

Extrinsic motivation – that is, the motivation that comes from outside of ourselves like friends and family – is usually limited because it can't always be there when we need it. It's easy to feel discouraged if you don't get any encouragement from others or if you feel like no one really understands what you're going through. You need to find your own source of intrinsic motivation – a reason for yourself to want to change and lose weight for yourself – to help keep yourself on the straight-and-narrow.

Your support system will keep you accountable to your goals. To keep going, you need the assurance that if you fall off the wagon, your friends and family will be there to help you get back on track.

People who have a strong support system can find it a lot harder to fall back to their old lifestyle because they don't want to disappoint others. They want to prove that they can do it. If a member of your support system falls off the wagon, encourage them to get back on track and remind them that they have the support of everyone around them.

Using affirmations to turn negative body weight thoughts into positive ones. Affirmations are positive statements that we repeat to ourselves in order to change our thoughts and beliefs. These words help us focus on what we want (a healthy body), feel good about ourselves, and give us the motivation we need to stick with our goals. Affirmations can be used alone, or they can be used in conjunction with a lifestyle change.

The subconscious mind is quite powerful, and we tend to internalize negative messages that we hear over and over again. In an effort to combat this, affirmations can be used in conjunction with a lifestyle change. Affirmations are used to help us change our negative internal monologue into a positive one by turning these negative messages into positive affirmations and making them the main focus of our day.

Affirmations are positive statements that we repeat in order to change our thoughts and beliefs. These words help us focus on what we want, feel good about ourselves, and give us the motivation we need to stick with our goals.

**How can we use affirmations to help us reach our goals?**

It's simple. We need to change our internal monologue from negative thoughts about body weight and turn them into positive affirmations.

For example, instead of telling yourself that you are fat, tell yourself that you are in control of your body weight and that you will not eat one more piece of cake today. Make this a positive affirmation because it is a positive statement about your life.

Another example if someone says to us "You're too fat." Instead of telling yourself "Oh no! I'm too fat. I'm going to pack on even more pounds" instead repeat a positive affirmation. Tell yourself "People are rude. I would never say that to someone else." This is a true statement about you, your beliefs, and your actions. Never allow another person's words to define you and make you feel bad about yourself.

Instead of telling yourself that you are unhappy with your body weight, tell yourself that "I enjoy exercising and eating healthy foods." This is positive because it is what one chooses to do with their life. Another example, instead of telling yourself that you're too ugly, tell yourself "I am beautiful." This will help you believe in your beauty and enhance your feelings of self-worth. A positive affirmation will help you feel better about yourself and believe in yourself and your body weight.

Affirmations are great because they help us change and reframe the way we view ourselves and the way that the world perceives us. It's all about what we choose to believe and internalize. Therefore, we must be careful not to overindulge in negative affirmations or allow others to control our lives through their words.

The key to using affirmations effectively is to simply repeat a positive, empowering affirmation - one that you want in your life- to yourself daily, as often as you can.

You will begin to notice a shift in how you think, feel and act as soon as you start using self-affirming affirmations. You will begin to believe that everything is going to work out for you.

**Putting it all together**

The goal of this exercise is to identify the core and dominant messages that you hear most when you are in conflict. Through this exercise, you will begin to understand the messages you are sending yourself and how they affect your feelings of self-worth and confidence.

For a week or two, I want you to pay close attention to your self-talk. The best way to do this is to keep a little notebook handy and write down anything you say to yourself. Make sure that you capture all the messages - kind, mean, or neutral.

Also, try not to avoid or repress any of the messages that pop up but rather try to be mindful of them and open in receiving them. None of these thoughts are "bad" - they are just messages!

When you have identified at least five main messages, identify the ones that you want to challenge. Write those down in a separate list and give each a number ranked in order of importance: 1 being the most important message and 5 being a less important one.

After you have ranked the importance of the messages, you will want to challenge them on the list. The easiest way to do this is to create a mantra for each message that is opposite of it. For example, if your main message number one is "you're not good enough," then you can counter that by creating a mantra around feeling special or adequate. Something like "I am enough" or "I am special." You can also write other statements such as "I am confident" or whatever feels comfortable for you. It's important to find a statement that feels right and works for you rather than just something generic.

Statements like "I am a good person" or "I am worthy" can also work well for this purpose. You may find that some of the statements you used on your list may not work as perfectly as others. That's okay - just keep going with the one that feels right to you!

When you have created a mantra and/or counter-mantra, write it down. In addition, write down the statements that you used to create your mantra.

The art of this exercise is to find a mantra that feels personal to you. This is not the exact mantra you will use when you are in conflict - this is simply for you to identify the negative messages that are most dominant in your self-talk and how to counter them.

This exercise will take some time. It may take a week or two to complete, but you will know that you are moving in the right direction when you begin to identify which messages are the strongest and how mantras that work for you will boost your self-confidence in dealing with conflict.

The goal is to find which messages are the most dominant in your self-talk, challenge them, and then construct a mantra to counter them. It's a simple process that will reinforce you belief in your own strength and ability.

# CHAPTER 4

# Set for success

We can all benefit from a little extra motivation when we are trying to achieve a goal. Getting motivated is a key factor to success: it's as important a part of the process as understanding what we're working towards. But what exactly is motivation?

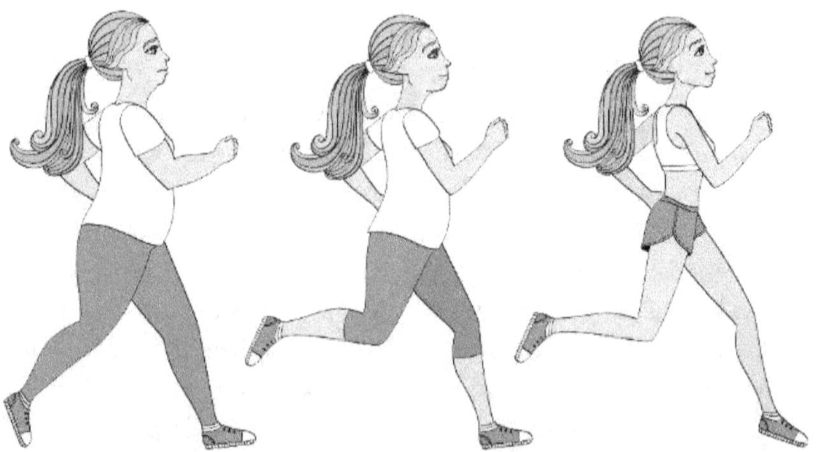

If you ask ten people what it means, you'll get ten different answers. They might say:

- "I don't like how I look in the mirror."

- "I want to have more energy."

- "I want to lose weight."

- "I want to feel better about myself."

- "I want my life to be easier."

61

- "I want to feel attractive and sexy again."

- "I want to be more fit."

- "I want to build my confidence."

- "I want to feel more confident with my body."

- " I want to feel powerful and in control of my life again."

- "I just want to be happy and enjoy life again."

There's a common theme here. No matter what anyone else says, the answers come back to a version of "I want to feel better about myself." This is what drives us. It's what we need. It's what we desire. Weight loss is all about becoming the best version of ourselves. In this chapter, we're going to see how you can find your "Why." This will be your focus for motivation, and it will give you the best chance to create a successful weight loss plan. On those dark days when you won't have the motivation to get out of bed, this will be your source of strength. When you're feeling down and fed up, this is the thing that helps you get back on track. On those days when you feel like giving up because things are tough, think about why you decided to start this in the first place. It's not just something that happened to you - it's something that was done to you and done with purpose. This is a powerful motivator - what we're looking at here is probably the most powerful force in all of nature: our purpose and desire for self-improvement.

**Let's take a closer look at what purpose actually means.**

Purpose is the driving force behind what we do. It's the reason why we decide to get up in the morning and go to work - simply because we have a purpose to fulfill there. Purpose is what drives us to be better, stronger, and smarter people. It is what drives us to continue with our education after high school, even if it means that we have to go into debt for it. Our desire for a better future for ourselves or for our children or our family drives us on every single day.

If you're frustrated with your weight loss thus far, chances are you're also frustrated with your life in general at some level. This does not mean that you don't like your life - quite the opposite. It means that you've realized that there's room for improvement. You're not where you want to be, and weight loss is what you have identified as your key to changing that.

This is where the power of your purpose comes in. What are your goals? Your dreams? What do you want to achieve? What do you hope for? If we can find a way to incorporate these things into our life, we'll always find a reason for getting up in the morning and looking forward to each day as it comes. The ultimate goal here is to create a vision or picture of what you want and how it will help you live your daily life better.

**Finding your why**

This is a soul-searching exercise where you'll unlock the answers and find the motivation you need. You need to think about why you got started with this in the first place. What led you to lose your weight? Take out a pen and paper and get ready to write down some things.

We're going to start with a very basic exercise here. You're going to think about health, career, finances, relationships, whatever is important in your life right now. Start writing down all the things that are important to you right now in your life - write everything down on the paper. Once you have completed this list, look at it again.


## Question 1: Why do you want to lose weight?

Maybe you've realized that going up the stairs isn't easy anymore. Maybe you've noticed that your clothes don't fit you anymore and if you don't do something about it, you'll start looking terrible. Maybe you're starting to notice that you're starting to put on weight again and you know that it's not healthy. Whatever the reason, just keep writing down all the things that are important in your life right now.


73% of Americans want to lose weight so that they can be healthier. If you're reading this book and saying, "I want to lose weight for my health," then this is the first place to start. The question we want to ask ourselves is:


"Why do I want to be healthier?" Maybe you're overweight because you lack exercise. Maybe you don't like the fact that your knees hurt whenever you walk up the stairs. Maybe you'd like to have a better vision or hearing. Maybe on another level, it means that it will be easier for you to get a job or help others in a professional way. Whatever it is, this should eventually connect with your purpose and give a bigger, lifetime perspective than just wanting to lose weight temporarily.


## Question 2: What motivates you?

What was the turning point when you realized that losing weight was the right thing to do? Maybe you saw a picture of yourself in a swimsuit and realized that you didn't want to be that person all your life. Maybe you saw an old friend and realized that they looked better than they used to and it motivated you to start losing weight. Maybe you were forced into changing your lifestyle because of a health scare. Whatever the reason, write that down into your "Why" list. Being overweight increases the risk of pregnancy complications, worse health, high blood pressure, and even heart disease. The reason you want to lose weight is to improve your health - it's the answer we should be looking at here. What do you think causes all these problems? What do you think causes premature death?

## Question 3: What will change after you lose weight?

This is a tough question - you obviously want to lose weight because you want to change something about yourself. What kind of change do you hope for? If you're married, do you hope that your bedroom life will improve? Do you hope to improve your career and become a better provider for your family? Whatever it is, get a pen and paper out and write down some answers. The question we ask ourselves here is: "What are the things that I'm hoping to achieve or improve?"

When most people think about their weight loss goals, they usually just think of "I want to lose weight" - that's not enough. It's very important to think about these goals in terms of what will change in your life once you've reached them.

The second thing we need to do is connect both things we've just learned - our **"Why"** and our **"What"**. Write down

65

everything you've learned in your journal. Make a copy of it, print it out, and do whatever you feel comfortable with. This is the step where you'll be able to find your own personal vision - your own personal purpose for losing weight. When you're done with that, read it over and look at the questions.

## Short-term and long-term fitness goals

A great way to keep yourself motivated is to set up some short-term goals. For long-term weight loss, 5% of your body weight per month is a good target. If you lose 5 pounds per month, that's 60 pounds in a year. That might be too fast for some people, so adjust it according to your fitness level and diet plan. Once you've found that target weight, break it down into smaller chunks - maybe 2% per week so that you're losing one pound of fat each week. Once you set up these tiny goals, you'll be able to find a reason for going to the gym every day or sticking to your diet plan.

Breaking down large goals into smaller, attainable steps is a key to long-term weight loss. The big goal here is to reach or improve your health, so you'll want to set up goals that are easy enough for you to maintain if that future condition changes. You'll also want to set these goals so that you hit them every week, so that you're meeting your short-term fitness goals on a regular basis. If you meet your short-term goals, then it will be easier for you to keep meeting them in the long term.If this is only an intermediate-level plan, then the focus should be on achieving the necessary fitness and nutrition levels that will help reduce your risk of diseases related solely to body weight.

Short-term goals may include things like:

- Being able to do a 20-minute workout at the gym

- Increasing your number of pushups

- Being able to eat 100 calories worth of healthy foods

 - Building up your strength by lifting heavier weights

- Keeping a food journal so that you can see what you're eating and how much of it.

Once you've achieved your short-term goals, put the challenges into your journal and keep track of them.  If you're losing weight - great! If not, try to find the reasons why this happened.  Maybe you were traveling and couldn't find time to exercise.  Maybe you weren't eating enough calories.  Whatever the case, keep track of these things so that you can get back to your goals in the future.

Finally, look at your long-term goals and how realistic they are.  Start by pretending that you've achieved your short-term goals and now want to lose weight for the rest of your life - what kind of results would you expect? It's really important for this question to be answered in terms of a "perfect world" scenario.  Why? Because once you've hit those goals, you'll want to do even better next time.

Long-term goals could include things like:

- Being able to do a 60 minute workout at the gym

- Taking part in a 10 mile run.

- Keeping a food journal so that you can see what you're eating and how much of it. This gives you the opportunity to change your diet in the future if necessary.

- Reading nutrition labels so that you know what you're getting into when eating a particular food. You might need more protein or more vegetables than usual when trying new foods, so it's important to know what they are.

## Tracking your progress

How will you know that you're getting the right results? That's what a fitness journal is for. It gives you an opportunity to keep track of your weight loss, so that you can see how it's changing over time. It takes some work to get going, but it pays off in the long run. You'll be able to see how much progress you've made and what steps you need to take in order to achieve your goals - if something isn't working well, then you'll know about it! Even if your weight loss is slow for some reason, the journal will show you exactly how much progress you've made. These are the metrics that you'll be keeping track of in your journal.

## - Weight

Weighing yourself is one of the most important things that you can do. It gives you an opportunity to consistently assess how much weight you're losing each week, so that you'll know if your diet plan is working. You'll also be able to watch the number on the scale go down as more weight comes off and down as pounds are lost.

- BMI - BMI stands for Body Mass Index, which shows us if we're obese or not.  It's a ratio - comparing your weight to your BMI in order to see if you're obese or not. BMI values for adults range from 18.5 - 24.9, so at a minimum, it's a good idea to keep this value in mind when you're tracking your weight loss.

## - Waist measurements

This one involves wearing an adjustable tape measure around your waist.

## - Meal records

This is where you track the number of calories that you eat at each meal and snacks throughout the day.  These should include the correct number of total calories, as well as all your other food groups that are essential for healthy living.

## - Fitness journal

The main thing here is writing down what you're eating, when, and how much.

## The non-quantifiable metrics

Your weight, BMI, waist circumference etc. are all very easy to track. They don't matter as much as you might think, though. These are the things that you should be focusing on:

## - How you sleep

We tend to fall asleep faster and sleep more soundly when we're losing weight, but it often means that you need more sleep in order to feel refreshed in the morning. Sleep is extremely important for weight loss. That's because your body goes into "repair" mode while you're sleeping, which increases the rate at which your metabolism functions during the day. That means that you'll be able to burn more calories, even when at rest.

**- Your mood**

This is also related to health, so it's good to know if your mental state is improving over time. It's important that you keep track of how you're feeling overall - and for this one, it might be a good idea to try writing things down every day compared with just once a week or every month. Are you stressed or anxious? Are you satisfied with your life? Are you sad at all? Are you happy, angry, bored, or frustrated?

**- Your energy levels**

As you start to exercise, and eat healthier foods, you will notice that you feel more energetic. You'll have more energy to do the things that you want to do, which will in turn help you lose weight. You'll be able to wake up earlier and exercise more often, which will be a real boost to your weight loss efforts.

**- Your sex drive**

This one will vary for everyone, but many people have found that their sex drive has increased as they continue to exercise regularly. It's not something you can measure with any accuracy, but it's still a good sign that you're getting healthier overall. Testosterone levels are higher in men who exercise regularly -

and for women, the sex hormones tend to increase.  What does that mean?  That means you're more likely to get aroused and more likely to enjoy sex.  Hormones don't lie!

## - How often you feel hungry

Hunger comes in two flavors - physical hunger, which involves your stomach growling and everything else associated with that feeling.  Then there's emotional hunger, which is when you feel the need to "nibble" all day long in order to stay satisfied. Keep track of both.

## When habits work for us

An interesting thing occurs when we follow the same routine for 21 days: We become more efficient. We are also more motivated, by our experience of succeeding at such repetition: In this case we derive from it such satisfaction that we make similar attempts again in the future.

The secret to improving your fitness is to not focus on losing weight - and don't worry about your weight loss rate either. Instead, focus on making healthy choices consistently and be patient with yourself while you change.

We'll do this by adopting healthy habits that will help us lose weight over time.  We already have the desire, so all we need to do is to make it a habit.

## Habits can be broken down into three steps:

- **Trigger** - The trigger is the event that starts your habit chain. It can be a specific thing, like smelling or tasting food, or something more abstract like an emotion or memory.

- **Routine** - The routine is the actual behavior that you'll be performing when completing your habit loop. This is what makes it a "habit".

- **Reward** - The reward is what you expect to get out of performing your habit. The reward is what motivates you to perform the routine over again.

The best way to stick to a routine is by understanding how the reward feels and deciding if you're willing to repeat it. If you feel good about performing the routine, then you'll want to repeat it. It's not that hard, really: It's all about reward.

## A morning routine

Mornings are the best time to start any new behavior - your brain is still at rest and you're not likely to be distracted. When we start the day by thinking of our fitness goals, we're more likely to resist temptation. Here are a few morning habits for weight loss that you can we'll start with.

- **Drink a glass of water.**

Drinking water in the morning will help wake you up and it also has some other benefits: It will help flush out your liver; it'll hydrate your muscles so that they'll be more likely to burn fat rather than carbohydrates; and it will keep your kidneys clear, which will make sure that your body is properly processing all fluids. Water is important for your health, so make sure to keep it at the front of your mind every morning.

During the night, your body's muscles break down glycogen, a type of carbohydrate stored in your muscles as energy. This is why your muscles have the appearance of being smaller when you wake up. Drinking water in the morning will help flush out what's left of this glycogen so that it can be used by the rest of the body.

- **Meditate for 10-15 minutes each morning.**

This can help your mental and physical state overall, aiding in your mood and productivity throughout the day. It also helps with a lot of other things: It improves focus, reduces stress, and even improves memory retention. It's not just helpful for weight loss by itself, either - it'll boost your health over time as well!

Before you get out of bed, close your eyes and take a few slow, deep breaths. Breathe in through your nose and breathe out through your mouth. Focus on your breathing and try to clear your mind of any thoughts.

- **Work out for 15-30 minutes each morning.**

A quick exercise session can be a wonderful way to start the day. It'll get you moving around, and it will wake you up mentally as well, which is perfect if you have a hard time getting up early in the morning. Exercise doesn't have to be long - it just has to be enough to make you feel good about it!

73

Jumping jacks and pushups are two great exercises that you can do.  You can do a quick session of each one, or you can mix them up. You can also run for 30 minutes or so if you enjoy running.


- **Make a meal plan and eat it - breakfast included**

There's something really motivating about knowing what you're going to have for dinner later in the day. It's even better if you know that you must cook dinner yourself! By creating a meal plan, you will be more likely to stick with your diet and lose weight. Also, making a detailed meal plan will help you figure out exactly what to do with your calories in order to meet your weight loss goals.


## Be mindful

Mindfulness is a relatively new term, although it's been around for a long time. Essentially it means being aware of your mind, body, and surroundings.  For instance, when you're driving, you should focus on what you're doing at the moment. Avoid your phone from lighting up with Facebook notifications or texts, instead, focus on the road! If you can't help yourself from getting distracted by those notifications, then put YouTube videos on the other side of the car dashboard so that you won't watch them while driving.


Remember to notice when you get cravings. Just notice them, and then take deep breaths to calm yourself down. Don't let your mind get worked up into a frenzy. Mindfulness is a great technique that can work wonders in your life.  It's healthy and it's also fun!

If you want to succeed at weight loss, you're going to have to start working on it every day. You're going to have to make exercise and eating right into habits that you'll keep for life.

**Healthier choices on autopilot**

Many fitness decisions, like choosing to have a salad instead of fries for lunch, can be difficult to stick to. The reward you're going to get from eating a salad is bigger for sure, but there's something about fries that makes them more attractive. The fries will give you immediate satisfaction and pleasure, while the salad won't be as good in the moment. If you want to lose weight, you're going to have to work hard with your self-control every day! There are a few things that we can do to make it easier for us to follow through with our plan.

Our willpower is finite. It gets used up throughout the day, especially when we make decisions. If you spend all day making good choices, then you'll likely lose your willpower by dinner time and give in to what's convenient (like a bag of chips). There are a few things you can do to counter this:

Firstly, make it as easy as possible to stick with your plan. If you make it too hard to do something healthy, like driving far away to the best grocery store in town or preparing gourmet meals from scratch every night, then you're going to be more likely to give up on it. That's why practicality is important! If it's too hard, then you won't follow through.

For weight loss, this means planning ahead and making sure that you have healthy food in the house.  If your pantry is filled with junk food and high-calorie meals that are easy to prepare, then you're going to be more likely to go for those. If your pantry is filled with special ingredients that are only used for recipes that take time, then you're less likely to try to cook them up and seek out a healthier substitute. After all, they'll just end up sitting there!

Having healthy food on hand makes it easier for us. Fruits and vegetables are obviously great for losing weight but having a few healthy snacks to tide you over throughout the day can also be helpful.  These could include things like nuts, seeds, and other ingredients that you're able to munch on throughout the day, without making anything healthier. There's no need to spend lots of money on these snacks either - a simple handful of nuts will do the trick!

Baking and roasting is better than frying. Fish, chicken, beef, pork, and vegetables will still taste great even when you cook them in the oven with no added fat from frying.

Another way to make it easier on yourself is to measure out portions.  Measure out how much food you'll be eating and then stick to that amount for the rest of the day, so that you won't go back for seconds. As a general rule, your stomach should be around 1/3 full when you finish eating your meals. When it's too full, your body will try to store any excess calories as fat and then build up more fat around your middle.

Consider replacing your favorite fast food with a restaurant. For instance, you could replace McDonald's with a Subway sandwich shop. Subway sandwiches are about the same price as Big Macs and they're packed with veggies and lean meats. You can make it even better by ordering double the veggies and double the meats instead of prying on the sauces for more flavor! In general, you want to eat smaller meals throughout the day. This way, you'll be less likely to overeat at any one sitting.

Again, this is a matter of practicality. It's very hard to eat less over the course of the day if your meals are huge. It's also very hard to eat less over the course of the day if you're starved by dinner time, since you'll be eating large portions so that your body has enough fuel to keep going until the next morning. By eating small amounts throughout the day and stopping before you get too full, you can lose weight and make it much easier on yourself at dinner time.

**Practicality triumphs willpower every day.**

Knowing that you can eat healthy at any time makes it easier for you to commit to changing your habits. By creating practical goals and making the process easier for yourself, you can easily stick to your plan. Planning out your meals is extremely helpful, but if you're not doing it then don't worry about it! It doesn't mean that the weight loss isn't going well - it just means that you're more likely to make the wrong choices when there's no planning involved.

**Our best chance to win the war on obesity**

You will face challenges on the road to success. To lose weight, you're going to have to overcome any habits that are holding you back.  For example, if there's a subway station near your house, then you're probably going to be tempted to buy a sandwich on a regular basis. If there are fast food restaurants near your office, then it can be hard not to fall back into the habit of grabbing a quick meal while running out the door in the morning.

If there's unhealthy food readily available in your neighborhood, then you're probably going to need some clever ways of making sure that you don't stray too far away from your plan. When we learn to anticipate challenges and find ways of combating them, even before they happen, then we can start to turn things around. By using our willpower to wisely anticipate the next challenge, we can cut down on the amount of willpower we will need to spend in the future.

**1.) Plan for a relapse**

It's inevitable that you'll at one point give in to temptation and fall off the wagon.

Once you've mastered your habits and made them second nature, you won't have to think about them as much.  It's a good idea to plan out what will happen if you do fall off the wagon. What will you do instead of eating unhealthy foods? How will you deal with that situation? Will you fall back to your old ways after giving in to deep fried chicken wings or chocolate cake? If so, how will you avoid giving in the next time? Having a strategy for a relapse goes a long way.

## 2.) What will you do when you won't have the time to cook a healthy meal?

This is an obstacle that you will face all the way along with the other excuses for giving in to temptation. Even if you planned out a strategy for when you don't have time to cook, it won't be enough. You're not going to have time to plan out your 30-minute healthy meal when your kids are screaming, the phone keeps ringing off the hook, and you're busy running from meeting to meeting.

Have an alternate strategy ready for this scenario: meal prepping in advance and freezing some healthy meals. Plan out what you want to make and how healthy it is. You can use this method even if you don't have time to cook anything at all. You can just pop a couple of meals in the microwave or put them in the oven while you're doing something else.

## 3.) You'll find exercise boring

People don't always make the right food choices because they don't have time. Another common reason people fall off the wagon is that they find it boring to exercise. That's why we have to find a new way of exercising that we enjoy doing while still working out those muscles. If you hate running, then try playing a sport instead. If you're afraid of lifting weights, try a boxing class for an alternative approach.

## 4.) You'll get bored eating the same thing over and over

Having trouble sticking to your diet? Are you feeling hungry because your diet is lacking flavor? It's not as easy as grabbing a burger on the way home today if you've been eating nothing but

79

salads all week long. Find a way to spice things up in the kitchen so that your diet is interesting, exciting, and not repetitive.  Just a few simple examples are using different types of spices and herbs, adding a twist of lemon juice or vinegar with some olive oil on salads, cooking up a batch of chicken fajitas with some extra guacamole on the side…you get the idea.

## 5.) You'll lack the time to go to the gym

This is for people who hate the gym.  The truth of the matter is that it can be very easy to latch onto an unhealthy habit like television if you don't have anything else to do. If you're busy all day, then trying to fit in a workout even at home while watching your favorite reality show won't be high on your priority list. Find a new way to exercise that you enjoy doing at home.  Maybe start with just taking a walk around the block or playing basketball at your local park after work.  No matter what, find something that's not too hard or boring, but still gives you some exercise with less effort than going to the gym and sweating it out in front of other people.

Swimming, riding a bicycle, and playing soccer are just a few examples of things you can do at home. Another option is doing some yoga at home, or if you're a big fan of dance music then try Zumba. You can exercise and dance at the same time, which is something that we couldn't do in the 1990s' with much success...

## Learning and appreciating your body

As time goes by, you will become more aware of your body and how it looks.  You will become more sensitive to the feelings that you have during different times in your day.  Your muscles will start to feel stronger, your skin will start to glow, and you'll start to see a bit of muscle definition.  It's important to appreciate these changes in yourself and not have a big reaction every time you see them. This can be as easy as taking a walk through the mall or sitting on the park bench, enjoying the feeling of the breeze on your face, and watching people around you go about their day.

You will know what healthy foods are cheaper and more affordable in your area, and which stores and restaurants offer the cheapest meals.  You will have set aside time to cook a healthy meal even when you're busy with other things. You'll have a strategy to carry out when you give into temptation, fall off the wagon, or lack the time or energy to exercise. You'll be able to see results from your hard work, not only on your health but on how well you look as well.

After 3 months of working at it, you'll be able to enjoy the fruits of your labor and succeed in your quest for weight loss. You will have learned your body and what it needs to be satisfied and healthy. You might even have lost a few pounds without even realizing it or built a little muscle that you can flex at the beach next summer. They say that weight loss comes from the combination of diet and exercise.  That's why it's important to keep track of your exercise progress in order for your health plan to work.

# CHAPTER 5

# A tough mental core

In sales, 80% of prospects say "No!" 4 times before they say "Yes!". In dating, 69% of men get rejected in some way before the lady finally says "Yes!" to a date. In careers, it takes 10 to 20 job applications before you're invited to an interview. I'm sure you're starting to see a common theme here.

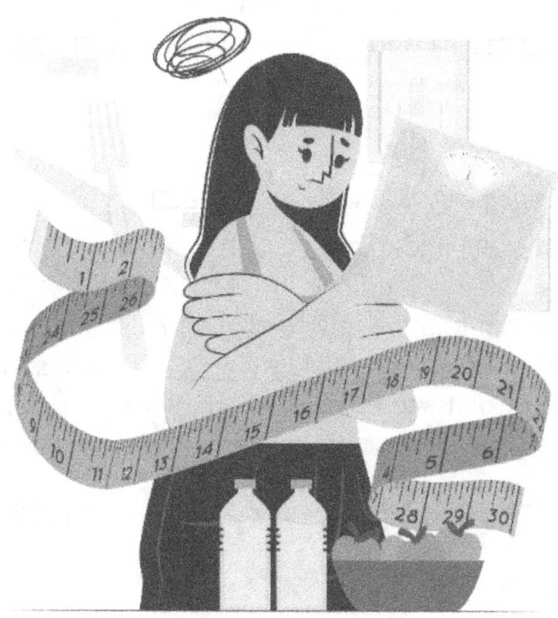

The odds are stacked against us, but there's something we can do about it. Over the course of our lives, we need to build a tough mental core that's able to bounce back from rejection, failure, or other obstacles that occur in our lives. Otherwise, we're going to fall back into our old habits and succumb to all the dangerous temptations of life.

When it comes to adopting healthy habits, it can be tough to make it stick. You have to make eating healthy delicious, which is not as easy as throwing a salad on the dinner table. You have to get up early and exercise even when you don't feel like it. In this chapter, we're going to learn about a unique technique for overcoming obstacles and relentlessly pursuing sustainable habits.

**The obstacles you'll face**

- Cravings for unhealthy foods

You're trying to eat healthier and lose weight, but then you see a group of friends eating pizza at the mall after work. You long for that salty pizza, the crunchy pepperoni, or that oozing cheese. What are you going to do about it? Are you going to give in and go find one of those pizzas for yourself? Is it easier just to skip dinner altogether so you don't have to fight that craving? When some people face this situation, they will succumb to temptation. They will give in and end up eating an entire pizza that night because they know they can't have any more pizza later on.

Freud's psychoanalytic theory offers one explanation for this type of behavior. He believed that every one of us goes through frustrations and developmental obstacles in life. We have an unconscious type of energy that builds up in our mind and body, but we don't know how to deal with it appropriately. To deal with these frustrations we have to find some kind of way to release this energy, or else it will build up and become destructive. According to Freud, our id is the source of all these worst parts of ourselves. If we don't learn how to manage this energy properly as children, then we may not be able to manage it properly as adults and end up hurting ourselves or others.


- A busy lifestyle

How many hours do we have left after sleeping for 8, spending another 8 at work and doing the things we have to do? What about our families and hobbies? We have about 2 hours per day left for everything else that we want to do. Finding time to take a walk, or to run three miles at the park may be impossible for some people. It's important to establish a schedule and maybe a highlight of that day where you will exercise. You must break down exercise into inconsequential amounts, so you won't feel guilty if you skip out on one of these little sessions.


We make time for everything else in life, but we seem to find it hard to make time for ourselves. But what else do we have time for anyways? We have so little time when you break it down by the hour. If we don't make time for something, what are the consequences of that?


- Lack of commitment

Let's be honest, weight loss can be a tough job. We have to set aside time for exercise, planning, and eating healthy. Even if we're leaving work early and going to the gym (which is already hard enough), we'll have to stop by the store on our way home to pick up some healthy food. It just seems like there are too many steps involved in this process. We start off full of energy and enthusiasm but then we lose our motivation somewhere along the road. Then it's back to square one with all of those obstacles in front of us again.

We see this happen over and over again with weight loss programs everywhere: the number of steps in implementing the program is greater than the number of pounds you'll lose by implementing it correctly.

Willpower is very limited. It is a finite resource that will eventually expire. If you keep struggling with temptation and get too frustrated, then you'll start resisting the things that you know will make you healthier (like exercise). You'll succumb to all those temptations that are placed in front of your path (like eating unhealthy foods and eating when you're not hungry).

You must be persistent and stick to your plan no matter what happens, or else the weight loss program will fail. The key to getting results is through repetition and consistency. As soon as you become complacent in your diet, then all the work that you've done up until now can be wasted.

- Hitting a weight-loss plateau

You're finally starting to see the results that you've always wanted. You're eating healthy, exercising more, and seeing the pounds melt away. Then you get to a point where progress slows down. You're struggling to lose weight even after putting all your effort into it, and you feel like it's not worth it anymore. Some people will see this as the end of the road, and then they'll quit. The only problem is that they don't realize why there's a plateau. There are many reasons for a weight loss plateau, but there are also solutions for getting past this problem.

It starts with understanding that your body is fluctuating all the time, even if you don't feel like it's changing. The body has complex systems in place to regulate and stabilize itself. Every time you go on a diet, there are changes in hormone levels and chemical balances which prevent you from losing weight again. However, you're also creating new habits and lifestyle changes that will help support long-term weight loss. It takes time for these changes to take place, but eventually, they'll become permanent without much effort at all.

**Mental toughness: A secret weapon**

By definition,, mental toughness is the ability to persevere in situations where you might normally give up. Mental toughness is also when you are able to overcome difficult challenges and succeed despite your lack of skills or experience. You're already trying to get yourself healthier, so why not try to be mentally tough as well? Being mentally tough can help you achieve your weight loss goals faster than if you were aiming for a quick fix solution.

You will have obstacles throughout your weight loss journey, but if you stay focused and persistent then all these obstacles will become easier and less challenging for you.

Big changes have small beginnings. Grit and perseverance are the driving forces behind any successful weight loss program. Mental toughness will get you past the obstacles that you come across in life, especially those that make you feel like quitting. The key is to find a balance between wanting the results and putting in the work needed to achieve those goals. If you're able to do this, then there's no telling how far you can push yourself to achieve more.

In order to establish a weight loss goal that will last, it is important to have your mind and body in sync with one another. You need willpower, determination, goals, and belief in yourself to begin your journey toward a healthy lifestyle.

Adopting a winner's mindset starts by believing that you can achieve your goals. If you believe that you'll succeed, then your chances of succeeding are much higher. We can influence our own thoughts by taking the time to visualize how we want to be and what we want to accomplish. If you are someone who has a hard time believing in yourself and your work, then it's important for you to take small steps towards achieving your goals.

Hyper-focusing on the task at hand is something that helps with the mental toughness aspect of a weight loss program. By putting all your energy and focus into the task at hand, you are more likely to succeed and stick to your plan. This is vital if you want to lose weight and keep it off forever.

It takes time for willpower to build up when fighting temptations towards unhealthy foods. At first, you don't have a lot of willpower to use for your goals, but you'll eventually get there by constantly pushing through these obstacles that come across your path. The difference between people who succeed in weight loss or don't succeed is how long they can hold out for.

**Building a tough mental core**

**I.)** It starts with adopting a growth mindset

How many times have you heard things like "you have to believe in yourself" or "believe that you can achieve it"? In reality, believing in yourself is what will help drive you toward your goals. Self-doubt will keep you from achieving any of your goals. This is why it's important for you to believe that you can achieve your goals and achieve them with ease.

It may be difficult to believe in yourself when you don't see results at first, but this is a sign that you're on the right track. Once you've started seeing results, then start believing in yourself even more. It's a positive feedback loop where you're continuously improving your ability to achieve goals. The more you do things that you're capable of, the more confident you'll become, and the more you'll believe that you can achieve great things in life.

**II.)** Then we have to change our view of obstacles

Obstacles aren't always bad. In fact, they can be a force for change and motivation. What is most important is how you manage them. You are only as good as what you can do in any given moment. Obstacles are often the things that are holding you back from achieving your goals or even from trying in the first place. So instead of looking at obstacles as something to avoid or get rid of, look at them as something that keeps you on your toes and engraves new patterns into your brain, so you become better and more resilient in the future.

Challenges are the way to change your life for the better, so make sure you keep pushing through all of them.

**III.)** Understand that it's OK to slip up once in a while

Let's say that you were at a party, and you ended up eating some fatty and greasy food. This is OK. It doesn't mean that you're a fat loser or that you have to feel guilty about what happened while you were out at the party. These things happen, but you now have the power to move on and do better in the future.

The more experiences we have with failure, the more chances we have of succeeding in life. It's all a matter of perspective and your thoughts about what happens to you during times when you feel like giving up. What's important is learning from your mistakes so you can improve for next time and make sure that these mistakes don't happen again anytime soon.

Don't give up after relapsing. Don't beat yourself up and focus on what you can do to improve next time.

**IV.)** Find a source of motivation

Everybody has something that motivates them to do well. Whether it's your family, friends, or a pet. The point is you have to find something that motivates you in order for you to feel inspired and confident enough to keep pushing forward with your weight loss program.

There are many different ways for you to develop mental toughness as well. You can do this by taking on difficult challenges and seeing how far you can go before things get too hard. If you're able to push through these feelings, then it will be much easier for you when trying to lose weight.

## Food for thought

If you've tried losing weight before, what challenges did you face? Did you find it difficult to stick to your diet or plan? How did you handle the challenges that came your way?

If these obstacles come up again, how will you overcome them? If you feel like giving up on your weight loss program, then what will help you get back on track?

What motivates you to push through these difficult times? Is there anything out there that will help keep you motivated and focused on reaching your weight loss goal?

We all know how hard it is to stay motivated with a diet. It's hard enough to think about eating healthy and nutritious meals for the rest of your life. It's even harder when thinking about the foods that we love most and the foods we think about whenever we're hungry. Though it's not easy, you need this mental toughness if you want to achieve success in the long run.

# CHAPTER 6

# Of food and nutrition

Can you outrun a poor diet by exercising like crazy? Researchers at the University of Sydney in Australia found out that irrespective of how much we exercise, eating right is still an important part of our health and wellness. This is why it's important to get informed on what we're eating and why it's so important to our health and vitality.

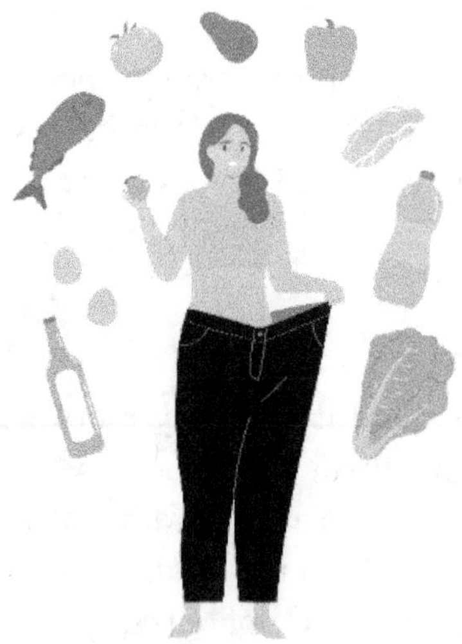

We live in a world where fast food is cheap, and we can purchase it anywhere. This makes it hard to eat healthy and nutritious foods that can help us lose weight. Nowadays, people are living longer because of medical advances, but at the same time, accessing unhealthy food is easier than ever. Delivery apps such as UberEats and JustEat make it easier for us to order anything we want. And all these unhealthy meals and snacks are usually much cheaper than the healthy ones.

People are spending less time cooking in the kitchen and more time eating out at restaurants, thanks to our busy schedules where we have less time to prepare healthy meals.

It's important to remember that when you go out to eat, you are responsible for everything that goes into your body. You can't blame food delivery services or restaurants for what you're eating.

**Why food still matters**

The importance of observing what we're eating and just how much we're consuming is still valid as this is a big part of maintaining a healthy lifestyle. When you think about it, we have immense control in what we eat. Being overweight is a result of eating the wrong kinds of food at the wrong kinds of times and this is the main reason why 40% of adults are overweight or obese in America.

Refined, simple carbohydrates such as grains and sugars spike blood sugar levels and over time, our internal organs become more insulin resistant which destroys muscle tissue and increases fat storage in our bodies. When you have excess fat around your waist, it's hard for you to burn fat due to four reasons.

**A.** Excess body fat leads to hormone imbalance that affects the way you process food and sugars in your body.

**B**. Eating simple carbohydrates will lead to insulin resistance which can cause weight gain, sleeping disorders, mood swings, anxiety and irritability.

**C.** Insulin makes more fat storage in the body and keeps your body from releasing the stored fat from other parts of the body.

**D**. When you eat sugar and simple carbohydrates, your blood sugar drops making you hungry and hungry makes people eat more food.

Here are a few benefits to healthy eating that you can enjoy every day.

## <u>We may live longer</u>

Life expectancy rates have dropped in the past 20 years and obesity is the main reason why this happens. Being overweight increases, your risk of many diseases including diabetes, heart disease, high blood pressure, and stroke. By eating more legumes, fewer processed meats, and less refined carbohydrates and sugars, you will have a much lower chance of contracting one of these illnesses.

The Mediterranean diet is one of the healthiest diets. It consists of high fruits, vegetables, whole grains, and healthy fats such as olive oil.

## <u>The right diet keeps the skin, teeth, and eyes healthy</u>

Have you ever noticed how fruits and vegetables are loaded with antioxidants that are good for the skin? Antioxidants help clean up free radicals released by the body which break down healthy cells in our bodies. Free radicals can also cause wrinkled skin, liver spots, and cataracts and even help cause cancer. The best way to battle free radicals is through a healthy diet rich in whole grains and fruits.

The eyes are one of our most important organs, but they are also one of the most sensitive parts of our body. By eating antioxidant rich foods such as fruits, nuts and dark greens, you can keep your eyes protected from common eye diseases like macular degeneration and blindness.

## - It's a way of boosting our immunity

Fruits and leafy green vegetables are loaded with disease-fighting antioxidants such as vitamin C and carotenoids, which boost the immune system. Eating foods that are rich in these vitamins and antioxidants, like fruits, apples, carrots and spinach will keep your immune system functioning properly which protects your body against infections.

## - Food is fuel for our bodies

We all know that energy is what powers our bodies to get things done. When we're out of energy at work or in school, we have to find a way to recharge so that we can keep going. Food is the biggest source of fuel for your body during the day especially when you exercise or do an intense activity like running a marathon.

Fats, proteins, and carbohydrates provide your body with the energy it needs to function at its best. When you eat foods that are rich in complex carbs such as whole grains, beans, fish, and lean meat, it provides energy in a slow and constant way that won't leave you feeling tired.

## - For stronger bones

As we age, our bones become more fragile and may break. When we eat a diet rich in calcium-rich foods like calcium-fortified soy milk, orange juice, green leafy vegetables, collard greens and almonds, our kidneys will be able to excrete the excess amounts of calcium in our bodies that forms stones in the kidneys. Eating foods with a high amount of calcium can also keep your bones strong and healthy.

## The 4 food groups

Most of us first came across the food pyramid when we were little kids, with the different food groups that came with a picture of a pyramid with them. Fats and processed sugars were at the top, meaning that we should only be having a small percentage of these in our daily diet, and the rest should be foods that were considered 'good' for us.

Below fats, we had the dairy group comprising of cheese, ghee, butter, yogurt, and milk. Then there was the whole grains group, which consisted of oats and wheat. As a result of these two basic food groups, the image depicted food in a very balanced way, giving us a healthy impression of what kinds of foods we should be having. From a young age we were taught that for us to be healthy we needed to give our bodies the right mix of fats, dairy, whole grains and so on. The practical application for the food pyramid today cannot be ignored especially when we need to lose weight.

## The kind of foods we should have in our diet

Dieting has become synonymous with losing weight, but this goal should be secondary to the real goal of good health. When we think of dieting, we should remember that it is not just one-dimensional. A healthy diet is all about balance and variety, so that our bodies are able to have the right kind of food at the right time. The fact of the matter is that when you start looking at it like this - thinking in terms of what kinds of foods actually suit us best and fuel our body with the right kinds of nutrients - then you start to see just how wrong it can be to label some foods as 'good' and others as 'bad'.

Even starchy foods that are labeled as "bad" like potatoes and grains are vital as they're the main energy source for our body. The amount of nutrients we can receive from certain foods is not just limited to nutrients such as protein, carbohydrates, and fats.

Vegetables like lettuce, Brussels sprouts, cauliflower, squash, and tomatoes are great sources of antioxidants that help rejuvenate the cells in our bodies. If you're looking to lose weight to improve your health, try having a balanced diet that is rich in fresh fruits and vegetables, lean meat or fish, and healthy low-fat dairy products like yogurt or cheese which provide essential vitamins and minerals for you.

Legumes, nuts, and seeds are also good sources of protein that have been linked to reducing the risk of heart disease. Supplements in your diet aren't always necessary and they can be quite expensive, so it makes sense to fill up on fresh foods that have more nutritional value than supplements.

Nutritional experts tend to agree that we should try eating a variety of fruits, vegetables, grains, and lean proteins instead of always thinking in terms of 'good' or 'bad' foods. What matters is how much you eat in moderation instead of how many calories you're consuming. Our bodies need fuel in the form of high-quality nutrition to keep us healthy and that is what our diets should be centered around.

You should try not to get too hung up on each and every nutritional label you read. They're often meant to confuse you instead of informing you and they don't tell the whole story anyway. What counts is how your body feels, so if you eat a variety of foods that are good for your health, then everything else will fall into place on its own.

**Several smaller meals; instead of a few large ones**

Managing portions is also important to keep your body running at its best. By keeping a smaller number of meals a day, you will not have to eat as much food in order to feel satisfied. The more often you eat foods that take up more space in your stomach, the longer it will take for them to leave your system and so you'll feel fuller for longer. Experiment with different portions and see what works for you by simply cutting down on the amount of food from one type of food or ingredients when planning your meals and snacks. You can even skip the dessert portion of some meals if it's not necessary for you to gain weight.

Vegetables rich in fiber like broccoli and spinach, whole grains like brown rice and beans will take much longer to digest after you've eaten them and so you'll be able to feel fuller for longer.

**Keeping sugars, salts and alcohol at bay**

When it comes to alcohol, moderate consumption is about one drink a day for women and two drinks for men. However, keep in mind that what may seem like a light drink could actually contain quite a lot of calories. One shot of whiskey contains 120 calories and so does one beer, so you need to be aware that even though you're not eating much at this particular moment in time, you could be storing up on the calories for later.

Diet soda is best if you want to cut down on sugar; however, going without any sweetened drinks altogether is the healthiest option – especially as diet sodas can still contain chemicals that are potentially harmful to your health in the long run.

**Healthy eating on autopilot**

In this section, I will share a few tips on how you can make it easier to eat a healthier diet on autopilot, without having to think about it too much. Let's start with a small fix with a big return.

❖ **Eat your greens first**

The key to eating healthy is, again, more greens. That doesn't mean you need to eat a salad for every meal. It does mean that the majority of your meals should consist of at least one serving of greens and add some variety with things like grilled chicken breast or grilled salmon with a little lemon juice (yes, I suggest adding lemon juice to your meats). You might not be able to directly add fruits and vegetables to everything you make but you can easily find meats and vegetables that are naturally low in fat or sodium. The key is looking for foods high in protein and low in sugar (or high in fiber!).

### ❖ Minimize fat in meat

Baking and grilling your meat is a great way to minimize the fat content in your meals. The only problem with this is that you may need to sacrifice some of the flavour by using marinades or spices when you bake or broil your food. You can still bake or grill your food but try to use less of the marinades and spices to do so.

### ❖ Add fruits and vegetables to meals

About 50-60% of your diet should consist of fruits and vegetables. There are a few specific types of fruit that you will want to include in your diet with all of the good nutrition that they provide. These include blueberries, raspberries, strawberries, blackberries, apples (preferably organic), oranges, and limes. Limes and lemons can add a lot of flavor to your meals and the citrus in them will help you to feel fuller faster. Apples, oranges, and limes are also great for digestion so adding them to your diet will promote healthy bowel movements.

### ❖ Focus on adding to, not subtracting from your meals

You can easily add more color and flavor to your meals by simply adding spices, juices, and sauces. Add more fruits or vegetables with every meal by chopping up some peppers, tomatoes, or onions. Use garlic for added flavor instead of salt and always opt for salsa or hot sauce instead of ketchup when possible.

### ❖ Make healthy swaps

Instead of using salt in your cooking, try using herbs and spices instead. You can easily add herbs and seasonings to everything that you make such as soups, stews, hot dogs, burgers, or wings. You can also use different types of oils such as olive oil, avocado oil, or coconut oil (although coconut oil is not suitable for all people).

If you love to drink soda or other carbonated beverages, try switching to some sparkling water instead. Most sparkling waters use artificial flavorings and sweeteners to ensure that they taste great so you can enjoy them without worrying about the calories in them.

## A Conclusion

In this chapter, I have shared with you what the best foods for weight loss are. I've also given you some tips on how to make it easier for yourself to get the nutrition that you need from your food, whether you're eating out or cooking in. You shouldn't be too strict about your diet but there will be a few things that you should keep as a priority in order to get all of the nutrients that your body needs and to feel more satiated after meals.

101

So, what exactly should we eat? Most foods fit into one of four categories – proteins, fruits, vegetables, and grains. It's important to include them all in your diet. After all, they're the building blocks of life.

Keep in mind that you don't need to feel hungry or deprived while trying to eat healthier. I've outlined some of the ways that you can make it easier to manage your diet while including some simple suggestions for foods that you can easily add to every meal and snack.

All of this will allow you to get the satisfaction that you need from your food without feeling overstuffed or bloated after every meal or snack. It's not about eating less – it's about eating more but eating healthily instead of overeating on unhealthy foods like processed snacks and fast food.

# CHAPTER 7

## As we age

As we get older, our bodies begin to slow down. Our metabolism slows down and we don't tend to move as much as we used to. People who are more sedentary are more likely to gain weight as they get older because their metabolism isn't burning energy at a pace that it once did.

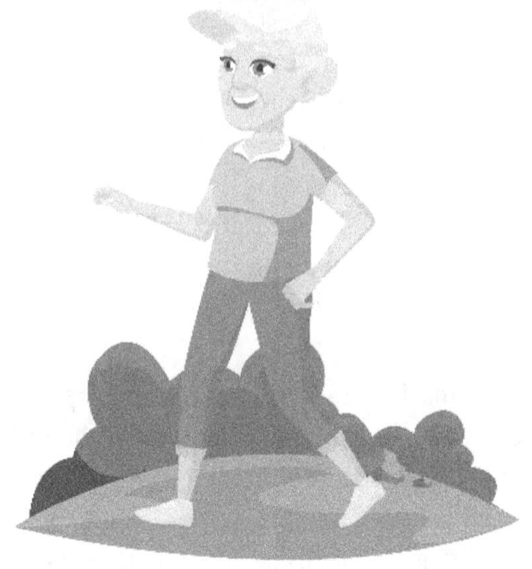

That doesn't mean that all seniors will gain weight or put on fat but it does mean that certain precautions need to be taken into consideration when the time comes.

Our bodies also begin to store more fat, especially around the abdominal area. The reason is that the muscles beneath our skin begin to atrophy as we age. We may not notice this process as we age but our bodies do. This means that we need to change some of the things that we eat in order to maintain a healthy weight in this area.

Women will also begin to experience menopause. and at this stage in life, their hormone levels change. These hormonal levels can also affect how much energy we use as well as how full we are.

**Why seniors have different dietary requirements**

Seniors need to eat different for two reasons. First and obviously, they don't need as many calories. Comparing the daily recommended intake of calories between a 45-year-old and a 75-year-old, you will notice that the 75-year-old only needs to eat 1,600 calories per day. This is considerably less than the 2,500 calories needed by the 45-year-old.

One of the reasons for this is because seniors tend to be less active than younger people. A lot of seniors spend long hours sitting down and not doing much. They might spend their days reading or watching television rather than going out and participating in physical activities like hiking or swimming. This is also why a lot of seniors tend to eat smaller portions throughout the day rather than three bigger meals (breakfast, lunch and dinner).

Secondly, underlying health conditions such as diabetes dictate the amount of food that seniors need. It's extremely important for seniors to have a healthy diet in order to control the progression of diabetes. This means that they need to eat less sugar and carbohydrates while increasing their intake of fruits, vegetables, and healthy proteins in order to balance out their blood sugar levels.

High blood pressure is another condition that seniors are more likely to develop as they age. Hypertension, which is the medical term for high blood pressure, puts you at risk of suffering from heart attack and stroke. Eating a healthy diet can help to reduce your blood pressure because it lowers your cholesterol levels and regulates the amount of sodium in your body.

These two factors (less food necessary per day and dealing with underlying health conditions) mean that seniors need to eat a slightly different diet than younger people. It's not as strict as a diet for someone with diabetes but it does have some limitations.

**The 4 diets that are recommended for seniors**

According to nutritionists, seniors who follow one of these four diets tend to live longer and have more fulfilling lives:

- The Dash Diet

- The Mediterranean Diet

- The Mayo Clinic Diet

- The Mind Diet

On the other hand, older people who follow a regular Western diet tend to feel more fatigued and have a lower quality of life.

105

This is because of the high levels of refined carbohydrates found in this type of diet.

## The DASH Diet

This diet is ideal for seniors who have high blood pressure and hypertension, which cause many cardiac and cerebrovascular problems. This diet forces you to consume foods that are rich in potassium and magnesium (potassium prevents water retention, while magnesium helps to lower blood pressure), as well as calcium and vitamin C. It can also reduce the risk of osteoporosis by eliminating foods rich in sodium (salt), such as processed meats, processed cheeses, high-fat dairy products, sweets, pastries; What's more, there is no limit on the amounts of fruits and vegetables you can eat. In this diet, you can eat white meat, poultry, fish, low-fat yogurt, and cheese; plus, you can include non-starchy vegetables such as:

- Broccoli

- Cucumbers

- Oranges

In this diet, you should not consume rice or white potatoes because they have a high glycemic index. You should also avoid eating high-fiber foods (like bread), which cause slow digestion that clogs the gut associated with your intestines.

## Why it works for seniors -

This diet stimulates the production of hormones that fight inflammation and keep your arteries healthy. It also improves digestion by enhancing hormone levels. Moreover, it is rich in nutrients that help to fight off diseases, such as cancer and Alzheimer's.

## The Mediterranean Diet

This diet, popular in the Mediterranean basin, is ideal for seniors because it has a low glycemic index. This diet consists of foods such as:

- Olive oil

- Whole grains

- Legumes (beans and peas)

- Fish (specifically oily fish)

- Fruit (mostly dried fruits and vegetables)

In this diet, you can eat white meat poultry, and fish. You should also include vegetables such as oranges, cucumbers, peppers, onions, garlic, leafy greens, and herbs. You can add nuts to your diet if you choose. You should avoid foods with high levels of saturated fats and carbohydrates that are rich in sugars.

In the Mediterranean basin, fresh fish, whole grains, and fruits are consumed regularly, which helps to improve memory and delay the onset of Alzheimer's disease and other forms of dementia.

## Why it works for seniors -

This diet helps to fight off depression by raising serotonin levels in the brain (serotonin improves sleep and reduces anxiety). It also combats inflammation and lowers inflammation-related disorders that affect seniors. The Mediterranean diet is rich in vitamins B6 (prevents heartburn), C (prevents scurvy) and K (prevents clots).

**The Mayo Clinic Diet**

Three meals a day, plus two snacks should be consumed, consisting of foods rich in fruits, vegetables, and whole grains. Alcohol should be consumed in moderation, while salt and sugars should be avoided.

In this diet, you can consume whole grains such as:

- Whole wheat bread

- Whole wheat pasta

- Brown rice

You can also eat vegetables and fruit. Vegans may choose to replace animal products with legumes (beans), tofu or nuts. In this case, the carbohydrate content of your diet may increase. You can also include soybeans (edamame) or use whole-grain products to prepare a faux tuna salad. Aim to consume at least 2 liters of water per day (1/2 liter for each meal).

The Mayo Clinic Diet is very rich in fiber, which prevents constipation and cancer. Your diet must also be low in saturated fat and sodium. In addition, you must consume a small amount of protein (about 1.2 grams per kilo body weight).

**Why it works for seniors -**

This diet helps to combat cardiovascular disease and cancer by decreasing inflammation, which affects the heart and arteries. This diet is also good for your brain because it contains high levels of omega-3 fatty acids (n-3 PUFAs), which enhance cognitive function in the elderly. In addition, this diet promotes regular bowel movements because it has a lower content of fat than regular diets.

At an age where people tend to complain about weight gain, the Mayo Clinic Diet allows you to lose weight, thanks to its low caloric content.

## The Mind Diet

This diet focuses on vegetables, fruits, nuts, and whole grains to stimulate your mind. You must also consume fish during this diet. This diet is rich in:

- Antioxidants (which stimulate brain function)

- Brain nutrients that slow cognitive aging (e.g., omega-3 fatty acids and vitamins B12 and E)

In this diet, you should avoid consuming alcohol because alcohol increases the risk of dementia. Martha Clare Morris, the researcher who started this diet, noticed that Alzheimer's disease was triggered by sugar and caffeine. Therefore, you should avoid sugar, refined carbohydrates and processed foods.

**Why it works for seniors -**

This diet improves sleep because it is rich in tryptophan, which slows down cognitive decline. In addition, this diet stimulates brain activity by increasing levels of biogenic AMPK (a molecule that increases energy in the brain). This diet also reduces inflammation that occurs in the brain and lungs (heartburn), due to its high fiber content. In this way, it helps to prevent heart disease and dementia by lowering blood pressure.

**Making mealtimes fun**

If your sense of smell (and taste) isn't as good as it used to be, experiment with different colors and textures.

With age, it's important to keep in mind that the sense of taste and smell fade. To compensate for this, try making mealtimes tasty and appealing by using colorful foods and unusual textures.

Put spices at the side of your plate or use complementary colors. Spices such as red pepper, turmeric, cumin and fennel as well as dark red fruits that have a strong flavor like plums, tomatoes can be used to give foods a more exciting taste. The same applies to complementary colors (e.g., blue foods and red fruits), which make you want to consume more food.

Textures are another way to add variety to the plate. For example, if the texture of a food is soft and smooth it is harder to chew, so try adding foods with a grainier texture. You can also add crunchy textures (e.g., nuts or croutons).

Aromatic herbs can also be added to your food, but you should avoid using too much. When cooking, look for herb flavors that are light and aromatic. This can be achieved by using fresh herbs or dried herbs. Asparagus, basil, and thyme are examples of aromatics.

You can spice up your meal with garlic and oil. Use a mild garlic flavor such as crushed garlic or pickled garlic if you're not a fan of stronger flavors.

## - Forget those empty calories

"Empty" calories is a fancy word for sugar and refined carbohydrates, which are foods that provide calories but no nutritional benefit. To avoid empty calories, you will need to reduce your portion sizes and limit the amount of sugar you consume. However, if you have a sweet tooth, there are healthier alternatives.

Sweet teas, sodas, desserts, and fruit juices can be high in sugar. If you are to have these, limit the amount you consume to one serving per day. To make your beverages healthier use fruit or vegetable juices that are unsweetened or add a natural sweetener such as honey instead of refined sugar.

## Mindful eating

With time, we learn to appreciate that there's more to meals than just the food on our plates. We see that a healthy meal can be an enjoyable experience in itself. Many of us also have come to appreciate the way food makes us feel full and energized or

111

nourished and relaxed. We've discovered that we can use this awareness in mindful eating to help us make healthy choices about what to eat and drink. Mindful eating means being aware of each sensory detail of food as it is eaten - sight, hearing, touch, smell, and taste. We are fully present with our food; we eat slowly to take pleasure from every bite; we stop when the first signal of feeling full is felt; we chew well to aid digestion; we enjoy our food instead of just eating it mindlessly.

Mindful eating is not a diet. It is not a set of rules, but rather an attitude we take to eating; it is a way of being in relation to what we eat. It means we are aware of our relationship with food and how food can be used as a tool for road-testing our responses and learning to appreciate what our body needs.

As you become more mindful, you will discover that you have more choices of overeating habits because you are less enslaved by habits that have taken over your relationship with food. You will find that your relationship with food becomes increasingly positive because the skill of mindful eating teaches us how to enjoy life's pleasures without feeling guilty afterward.

**Awareness is key**

Taking the time to become aware of even the subtlest details about what you are eating can make a huge difference to how you feel about your food.

To get started, start by being mindful of the journey you take when you eat. In doing this, you will learn to notice signs that signal the sensations of feeling full and needing to stop eating - especially a feeling of heaviness in your middle and stomach. Continue by being aware of the colors and sounds around you while eating. Encourage yourself to notice the taste and smell of your food, too - not only at first but as well throughout your meal.

The aroma of the food, taste, touch of food, and sight of it on your plate all have a role to play in mindful eating. All of them help you to stay present, focused, and full of enjoyment as you eat.

When you are done eating, take time to appreciate the flavors in your mouth and across your tongue, noticing how they change s the meal takes effect. Take some time to enjoy the sensations that come with swallowing, too - so that next time you can order your meal with confidence. By taking mindful bites instead of mindless ones, each and every mouthful becomes an occasion for heightened appreciation that opens up a new perspective on how we relate to food.

# CHAPTER 8

# Get moving

Can you outrun a bad diet? Let me phrase that differently. Can we eat as much junk food as we want and then try to burn off all the excess calories by exercising like crazy?

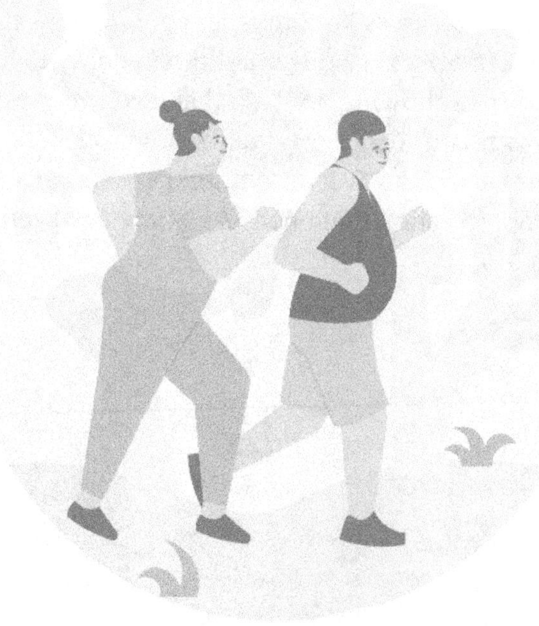

I think we all know the answer is no. Yet, we sabotage our fitness goals by making this very mistake. The truth is, getting healthy requires both a healthy diet and an exercise routine that targets all three of the components that make up our body.

You might have heard the saying, "Eat less, move more." It sounds like common sense, and it is actually the first thing your doctor tells you when you complain about being overweight or having high blood pressure. Exercise offers many benefits, including weight management and improved health. However, before you go running or jumping into an exercise program, make sure you know how much is enough to achieve your goals instead of failing miserably due to misinformation.

In this chapter, we're going to review some of the basics of exercise, diet, and some things you can do to improve the effectiveness of your efforts.

Let's start by illustrating why "exercise" and "working out" are two different concepts. Exercise refers to anything that gets your heart rate up. Working out is more methodological. Working out means the process of using your body to do something specific. This could be weight training, running, swimming, cycling or anything else that gets your heart pumping.

**Exercise is all about getting and keeping fit.**

Most of what we know about exercise is pretty much common sense; we've used our bodies for centuries for everything from hunting to manual labor to running away from wild animals and charging into battle.

115

**Why exercising doesn't always work for weight loss**

We overestimate the benefits of exercise when it comes to our waistlines. While we burn close to 300 calories during 30 minutes of moderate aerobic exercise, we typically overestimate the actual benefits. Most people have a hard time understanding that it's not actually possible to outrun a bad diet. Physiologically, it's impossible to burn more calories than you consume. We're metabolically programmed to match our energy output with energy intake, and this is a survival mechanism - after all, if we ate more than we needed, we'd store the excess as body fat.

Exercise accounts for only a small portion of daily calorie burn. To achieve weight loss, we need to vary our caloric expenditure by making healthier food choices.

Movement and physical activity can help with weight loss if done in conjunction with healthy eating and lifestyle changes. The most efficient way to burn calories is to make better food choices, but the best way to train your body to burn fat is through vigorous exercise.

A combination of both exercise and healthy eating can help those trying to lose weight reach their goal.

**Why we need to do it anyway**

Aren't we all familiar with the physical and mental benefits of exercise? We know that it boosts mood, improves self-esteem, and reduces stress. It can also improve your athletic performance and relieve symptoms of chronic back pain.

But for those of us who have time constraints, are injured or aren't athletically inclined, it can be challenging to find the motivation to get up and move. And it can be even more challenging to keep moving when you're not feeling that motivated.

This is especially true when things haven't been very good in your life lately. You might be dealing with increased stress or anxiety as a result of problems at work or at home, or maybe you're juggling a new job, new relationship and/or new baby while simultaneously trying to stay on top of household chores and other regular daily tasks.

The secret is not to rely on motivation alone. You need to have a plan in place to keep you not only motivated but doing what you have to do. Being proactive is key and the three steps outlined below will help you maintain that motivation.

**Step 1: Set goals.**

Set specific goals for yourself, as small as they may be. Even better, set a goal for where you want to be in six months and then set another goal for where you want to be in one year. Fitness goals should be closely linked to personal goals and shouldn't extend beyond your current physical capabilities.

**Step 2: Make a plan.**

The plan should include specific actions you can take to reach your goals. These actions could include exercise, meal planning, daily activities that support a healthy lifestyle, etc. It should cover all the bases so that you don't get discouraged when one area falls short of your expectations.

## Step 3: Follow the plan.

The third and final step is the hardest. This is where you need to make a daily commitment to follow the plan. Even when you don't feel like it, even when life gets in the way of progress - you need to keep going if you want to reach your goals.

## A little bit goes a long way

The most common recommendation for starting an exercise program is to gradually build up to 30 minutes of moderate-intensity exercise five times per week. Doing so, however, can lead people to expect immediate results that can be discouraging and lead them, once again, down the path of giving up and quitting.

## How it's tied to our attributes

The truth is that we've been looking at exercise from the perspective of aerobic capacity and endurance without paying enough attention to strength training. There are health benefits to having a high aerobic capacity, but strength is fundamental for optimal health. Muscular strength is very important in being able to do everything that we want to do.

Strength training improves balance, coordination, and agility. It can help improve your agility and power which will make you less likely to fall or get hurt if you fall.

In addition, muscular strength helps support your upper body so you have more energy available for other daily tasks that may require lifting. In fact, researchers have found that people who don't exercise regularly and lift weights are more likely to suffer injuries resulting from lifting groceries or doing yard work than those who perform regular weight-training exercises.

**The best exercise routine when you're in your 20s to 50s**

In this age group, aerobic exercises and weightlifting are important, but a combination of the two - also known as concurrent training - is recommended. This ensures that you are stimulating muscle growth and increasing lean muscle mass (which helps regulate body fat levels) while at the same time improving overall fitness.

A program that combines aerobic and resistance training three times a week, including warm-ups, cool-downs, and stretches, is ideal for maintaining a healthy body weight. The combination of weightlifting and cardio will also improve your ability to perform tasks of daily living. Squats, lunges, leg lifts ensure you stay flexible.

For those of you who are in your twenties and early thirties, you may need to incorporate more of a balanced program, including a combination of cardio and strength training.

Depending on your age, however, it's also important to keep in mind that muscle tissue tends to decrease more as we get older.

If you're over 40, it is recommended that you start strength training with lighter weights -- 25-30 pounds - to minimize the amount of muscle breakdown. This can be done on an alternating-set format and includes five sets per exercise: 1 - 5 reps for each set, resting 1-2 minutes between each set.

Exercising at this age range is about building lean muscle mass and ensuring that our weight-bearing joints are fit and healthy. It is also about keeping your heart and lungs healthy, so you should exercise for about 30 minutes per session. We're setting the foundation for when we get older.

**Working out at 60+**

If you're over 50, it is recommended that you choose an exercise that keeps your knees and hips in a more upright position. This may include squats and lunges rather than bent-over rows and shoulder presses. Do both heavy and lightweight exercises that are balanced to ensure muscular strength, and flexibility and improve overall health.

Stretching is also an important part of your exercise routine. It's as important as strength training and aerobic exercises.

As we get older, it's a good idea to increase our flexibility to improve balance, coordination, and agility so that we can do the same activities that we have always done when we were younger.

Plus, it's never too late to start exercising! Get out there and start moving, even if it is just walking around the block. No matter what your age is, you can still benefit from increasing your daily physical activity; not only will you look better but you will feel better about yourself too.

**Making exercise a part of you**

How do we find the time to incorporate exercise into our daily routine and how do we do it without having to give up on other priorities, like sleep? Here are a few tips to help you get started:

**- It starts by having a fitness plan**

Schedule workouts in the same way you schedule doctor's appointments and other activities. Planning a workout makes it more likely that you'll actually follow through and it will give you a sense of accomplishment.

If you'll be leaving work late on that day, fit in an after-work workout. You can fit in your workout during your commute and still make it to your child's soccer practice or a dinner date on time. You can even formulate an exercise plan that allows you to get out of the house and walk even on rainy days. All you need is an umbrella and some good, waterproof boots.

**- Exercise early in the day**

The earlier in the day you plan to exercise, the better. Find a time of day (early morning) when you are not overly tired and can focus on your workout. You will most likely be more energetic and focused at this time of day. Pushups and planks are great and easy exercises that you can do to get started. You don't have to buy a gym membership or even leave your home to do these.

This habit gives you so much more time in your day for other activities, and it also helps you become better at time management.

## - Use your commute to work as a workout

Riding the bike, walking, or running to work is a great way to get some exercise. Think of the time you spend commuting to and from work as a workout. You are still burning calories, but you are getting an endorphin rush at the same time because you're using your body for movement.

## - Use certain aspects of your daily routine to exercise

Using the stairs instead of an elevator or escalator or taking a walk around the block after dinner can make big differences in your overall health. When you're watching television, do some pushups while sitting on the couch. Home workouts don't have to be overwhelming and time-consuming.

# Conclusion

In this book, we've seen that losing weight and staying fit does not have to be complicated. We can make small lifestyle changes in our daily routines, and we will end up feeling healthier than ever before. Changing our bodies doesn't have to mean losing time from our day in order to exercise. There are simple activities that we can add into our lives, like taking the stairs or walking around the block after dinner, that will help us stay active while building lifelong habits that will be beneficial for a long time to come.

Throughout the book, we saw that a mindset shift is a large part of losing weight. If we want to improve our lives and our health, we have to change the way we feel about ourselves. Self-confidence is gained from knowing that we are taking care of ourselves. By eating healthy foods, exercising regularly, drinking plenty of water and getting enough sleep, it's no wonder that we will start feeling better about ourselves and even happier in general.

While making small changes in our daily routines may seem insignificant at first, they will add up over time. We will be amazed by how much better we feel as our bodies start to respond to these small habits. These habits will become part of our lives and living without them will become difficult to imagine.

The compounding effect is real. Small changes made over time will add up and become significant. If we start practicing these healthy habits now, we won't have to worry about making huge lifestyle changes later on in life when it's harder to focus on our health. If we can get into the habit of taking care of ourselves when we are younger, it will be easier to continue this routine as an adult.

If you find yourself struggling with weight loss, don't give up hope. It may not happen overnight, but you can make it work with a positive mindset and the right knowledge. Having a clear view of how weight loss works will help us stay motivated and focused on our goals until they're achieved.

# <u>Sharing is caring!</u>

Share this book with your friends and family on social media, or simply tell them about it. Sharing is the best way to get the word out and the best way to make a difference in people's life. Your effort will be appreciated by others who might be struggling with their health too, and they may find help in this book or your recommendation. The least you can do for others is to offer a helping hand, so please don't hesitate to share this book.

# A Request

125

If you've enjoyed this book, would you mind leaving a favorable review? It's greatly appreciated when you recommend this book to others, and every review helps spread the word. Thank you!

* 9 7 9 8 2 2 7 5 6 0 6 6 7 *